Symposium on

Ocular therapy

VOLUME FIVE

Symposium on

Ocular therapy

Under the auspices of the American Academy of Ophthalmology and Otolaryngology and the Association for Research in Vision and Ophthalmology

Edited by

IRVING H. LEOPOLD, M.D.

Professor and Chairman, Department of Ophthalmology, Mount Sinai School of Medicine, City University of New York, New York, New York

With 21 illustrations

THE C. V. MOSBY COMPANY

Saint Louis 1972

VOLUME FIVE

Printed in the United States of America

International Standard Book Number 0-8016-2956-X

Library of Congress Catalog Card Number 66-22972

Distributed in Great Britain by Henry Kimpton, London

Contributors

Leonard Apt, M.D.

Associate Professor of Ophthalmology, Department of Ophthalmology, Jules Stein Eye Institute, School of Medicine, University of California at Los Angeles, Los Angeles, California

Samuel B. Aronson, M.D.

Director, Eyetis Foundation; formerly Associate Professor in Residence, University of California, San Francisco, California

Bernard Becker, M.D.

Professor and Head, Department of Ophthalmology, Washington University School of Medicine, St. Louis, Missouri

Robert P. Burns, M.D.

Professor of Ophthalmology, John E. Weeks Institute for the Advancement of Ophthalmology, University of Oregon Medical School, Portland, Oregon

Philip P. Ellis, M.D.

Professor and Chairman, Division of Ophthalmology, University of Colorado, School of Medicine, Denver, Colorado

John E. Harris, M.D., Ph.D.

Professor and Head, Department of Ophthalmology, University of Minnesota Medical School, Minneapolis, Minnesota

Herbert E. Kaufman, M.D.

Professor and Chairman, Department of Ophthalmology, College of Medicine, University of Florida, Gainesville, Florida

Irving H. Leopold, M.D.

Professor and Chairman, Department of Ophthalmology, Mount Sinai School of Medicine, City University of New York, New York, New York

Theodore W. Lieberman, M.D.

Assistant Professor of Ophthalmology, Department of Ophthalmology, Mount Sinai School of Medicine, City University of New York, New York, New York

Thomas E. Moore, Jr., M.D.

Assistant Clinical Professor, Department of Ophthalmology, University of California, San Francisco, California

Steven M. Podos, M.D.

Assistant Professor, Department of Ophthalmology, Washington University School of Medicine, St. Louis, Missouri

Arthur L. Schwartz, M.D.

Assistant in Ophthalmology, Department of Ophthalmology, Mount Sinai School of Medicine, City University of New York, New York, New York

David Shoch, M.D., Ph.D.

Professor and Chairman, Department of Ophthalmology, Northwestern University Medical School, Chicago, Illinois

Frederick H. Theodore, M.D., F.A.C.S.

Clinical Professor of Ophthalmology, Mount Sinai School of Medicine; Attending Ophthalmic Surgeon and Director, External Disease and Infections Clinic, Manhattan Eye, Ear, and Throat Hospital, New York, New York

Vernon G. Wong, M.D.

Clinical Director, National Eye Institute, National Institutes of Health, Bethesda, Maryland

Preface

This publication records the information presented at the Drug Symposium of the American Academy of Ophthalmology and Otolaryngology and the Association for Research in Ophthalmology and Vision held as a joint meeting in Las Vegas on October 4, 1970. Each of the presentations is current and differs from those presented at earlier symposiums. As in preceding volumes, fresh information has been developed and also, as in the past, material has been kept to the fundamental and practical level. In certain areas information is included which was not as presented at the meeting, such as the chapter on inborn errors of metabolism, and the chapter on the management of intraocular infection has been revised.

Irving H. Leopold

Contents

Chapter 1 Management of inborn errors of metabolism with ocular involvement, 1
Irving H. Leopold, M.D., and Arthur L. Schwartz, M.D.

2 Toxicity of strong miotics in children with newer observations, 30
Leonard Apt, M.D.

3 Subconjunctival therapy, 36
Philip P. Ellis, M.D.

4 Virus therapy, 43
Herbert E. Kaufman, M.D.

5 Points in the treatment of bacterial corneal ulcers, 48
Frederick H. Theodore, M.D.

6 Plasma expanders and lytic agents in ophthalmology, 55
David Shoch, M.D., Ph.D.

7 Immunosuppressive agents in ophthalmology, 65
Vernon G. Wong, M.D.

8 Management and complications of systemic corticosteroid therapy, 70
John E. Harris, M.D., Ph.D.

9 Corticosteroids in infectious corneal disease, 77
Samuel B. Aronson, M.D., and Thomas E. Moore, Jr., M.D.

10 Intraocular pressure effects of diluted and new topical corticosteroids, 90
Steven M. Podos, M.D., and Bernard Becker, M.D.

11 Individual responsiveness to drugs and pharmacogenetics in ophthalmology, 96
Theodore W. Lieberman, M.D.

12 Effectiveness study of antibiotics, 105
Robert P. Burns, M.D.

13 Problems in the use of antibiotics, 113
Irving H. Leopold, M.D.

Symposium on

Ocular therapy

Chapter 1

Management of inborn errors of metabolism with ocular involvement

Irving H. Leopold, M.D. and Arthur L. Schwartz, M.D.

Up to the present time, about 50 conditions have been shown to have a basis in some form of inborn error of metabolism. In these conditions a block in a chain of chemical events within the cell permits accumulation of a toxic product or lack of an essential intermediate, and the effect of such a cellular disaster is hazardous to the host, often with widespread effects (Fig. 1-1).

Enzymes essential for body reactions are made of proteins and undergo continual renewal and turnover. This turnover is governed by normal principles of protein synthesis and demands a supply of amino acid building blocks, as well as a convenient energy source. This energy source is usually supplied by adenosine triphosphate (ATP). But

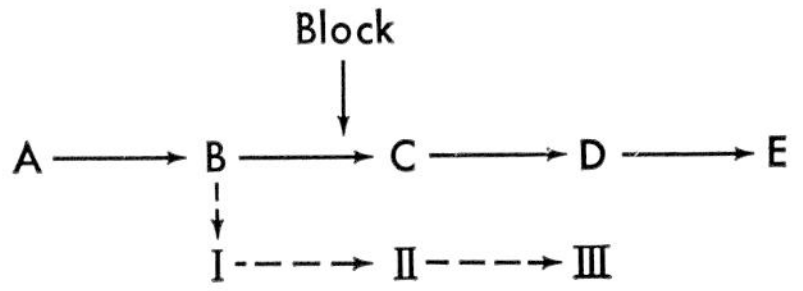

Fig. 1-1. Block in chain of chemical events within cell. The block may lead either to the accumulation of B, which may be toxic; to a lack of C or D, which may be essential for the health of the cell; or to an alternate route I, II, or III, which may be toxic.

the cell cannot produce a specific enzyme unless it first has proper direction from a genetic code involving messenger RNA and DNA.

Not all inborn errors of metabolism become manifest before birth or immediately after birth. Those involving enzymes that are not required by the fetus will not interfere with intrauterine development and may be amenable to postnatal therapy.

If the metabolic defect involves an enzyme that is required for the digestion of a nutrient, therapeutic success can be achieved either by making the enzyme available from exogenous sources or by providing an alternative nutrient. Both approaches have been employed successfully in treating dissacharidase and trypsinogen deficiencies.

If the inborn error involves metabolism of an essential nutrient for which there is no substitute, therapeutic success is less likely but still possible if the requirements for the nutrient can be met; but the amount of nutrient must be limited to a concentration low enough to avoid toxicity. This is possible, for example, in phenylketonuria (PKU) and disorders of protein metabolism that result in ammonia intoxication.

If toxicity results from the metabolism of an endogenously produced substance, limiting the exogenous source can at best be only partially effective.

An outline of the possible modes of therapy for inborn errors of metabolism is presented below.

A. Enzyme defects
   1. Reduce substrate
   2. Reduce substrate precursor
   3. Add product or its derivatives
   4. Add cofactor

B. Enzyme activity in excess: add substance that will reduce enzyme activity

Recently, considerable emphasis has been placed on prenatal and neonatal chemical diagnosis of inborn errors so that treatment can be initiated before irreversible damage develops. There is no doubt that such treatment may be effective. However, several factors should be considered.

Correction of the chemical abnormality will not alter the pathologic process if the basic defect that accounts for the chemical abnormality does not account for the clinical manifestations. For instance, cystathionuria and homocystinuria were first discovered during investigation of mentally retarded individuals. Every patient, therefore, was certain to be retarded, but it was far less certain that the retardation was causally related to the enzyme defect.

Even when both the clinical disturbance and the chemical abnormality are related to the same molecular defect, they may not be related to each other. For example, lowering the uric acid in the Lesch-Nyhan syndrome or the phytanic acid in Refsum's disease may not prevent or reverse the neurologic manifestations. The chemical abnormality most easily detectable may be irrelevant to the toxic process.

Although the chemical abnormality is related to the pathologic condition, the clinical manifestations may vary from patient to patient with the same defect; thus, a few patients in whom the classical signs did not develop have nevertheless been described as having galactosemia.

Discovery that the same metabolic reaction is blocked in several patients does not mean that the molecular defect or the treatment is the same for each. Some patients with methylmalonic acidemia respond to vitamin B_{12}, for example, while others do not.

The chemical abnormality may be transient, as in some infants with hyperphenylalinemia.

Even when the treatment is capable of preventing damage, the diet may be so stringent and different from normal that it produces disturbances. Some of the psychologic problems of children treated for galactosemia and PKU may be a consequence of the prolonged dietary restriction imposed on these children.

Our ignorance of the scope of the molecular variations and the nature of the disease-producing process in the inborn errors frequently makes preventive dietary therapy difficult to evaluate. The problem is compounded by the fact that a single investigator is unlikely to be able to follow a large number of patients with any one disorder.

The answer does not lie in abandoning screening programs for inborn errors in the newborn. If anything, screening programs have increased the knowledge concerning the variations of both the basic defects and the disease manifestations. Perhaps the answer lies in the establishment of prospective collaborative studies. It is obvious that we are still in the initial stages of describing and classifying inborn errors of metabolism, but some form of systematic evaluation of the clinical course and therapy of these disorders is still required.

Some of the major categories of inborn errors of metabolism with ocular manifestation are those of pigment metabolism, lipid metabolism, amino acid metabolism, and sugar metabolism. These disorders, outlined below, are some of the diseases to which the rest of this chapter is devoted.

I. Pigment metabolism
   A. Methemoglobinemia
   B. Sickle cell anemia
   C. Porphyrias
   D. Chediak-Higashi syndrome

- II. Lipid metabolism
  - A. Hand-Schüller-Christian (?)
  - B. Hereditary ataxic polyneuritis (Refsum's disease)
  - C. Lipid storage diseases
    1. Gaucher's
    2. Niemann-Pick
    3. Tay-Sachs
    4. Fabry's
    5. Lesch-Nyhan
- III. Changes in serum lipids
  - A. Essential hyperlipemia
  - B. Essential hypercholesterolemia
- IV. Amino acid metabolism
  - A. Phenylketonuria
  - B. Albinism
  - C. Homocystinuria
  - D. Alkaptonuria
  - E. Cystinosis
- V. Sugar metabolism
  - A. Galactosemia
  - B. Glycogen storage disease

PIGMENT METABOLISM

Porphyria

The porphyrins of the body are important in the formation of hemoproteins such as hemoglobin, myoglobin, and cytochrome oxidase, which function as carriers of oxygen in the blood and tissues. Porphyrins are produced as intermediaries or byproducts in the formation of hemoproteins from succinate and glycine. In this synthesis small amounts of uroporphyrin, coproporphyrin, and porphobilinogen (PBG) are found in the blood and excreted in the urine and feces. Most of the hemoproteins, catalases, peroxidases, cytochromes, and so on may be synthesized in any cell in the body. However, hemoglobin is synthesized only in hemopoietic organs.

There are several types of metabolic disorders of porphyrin metabolism. One of these is lead poisoning. In this disorder there is a block in the synthesis of hemoglobin from succinate and glycine. Increased amounts of coproporphyrin and amino levulinic acid are found in the urine. An elevated blood lead level establishes the diagnosis.

In hepatic disease such as cirrhosis, there is an increase of urine coproporphyrin; uroporphyrin may also be increased.

In porphyria erythropoietica there is an inborn defect in the conversion of PBG to uroporphyrin in the course of hemoglobin synthesis.

In addition, there is a marked overproduction of uroporphyrin. Thus, one finds large amounts of uroporphyrin in red cells, spleen, skin, and urine and feces.

In porphyria hepatica, acute intermittent type (AIP), there is a block in the conversion of PBG to uroporphyrin in the course of hemoprotein formation in the liver, with excessive production and excretion of porphobilinogen and delta amino levulinic acid (ALA) in the urine. In this disease the ALA synthetase activity is greatly increased.

The disease is transmitted as an autosomal dominant. AIP rarely presents clinically before puberty and may exist in latent form throughout life. The onset of symptoms is usually between puberty and age 30. Four factors have been demonstrated to be able to convert latent disease into active disease with neurologic dysfunction: certain drugs, sex hormones, infection, and starvation.

Drugs such as barbiturates, meprobamate (Miltown), chlordiazepoxide (Librium), griseofulvin, and sodium diphenylhydantoin (Dilantin) have been implicated in precipitating acute attacks.

Female sex hormones seem to play a role for a multitude of reasons: (1) the disease is predominantly found in women, (2) it appears clinically and biochemically after puberty, (3) some women with AIP have attacks that recur cyclically in relation to the menstrual cycle, (4) often there is an increase in activity during pregnancy, and (5) exogenous estrogen administration is able to precipitate clinical manifestations.

Diet plays a role because starvation increases symptoms, and increased carbohydrate intake has been shown to block the induction of hepatic ALA synthetase.

Clinically, severe abdominal pain is the most common symptom, and often the patient appears to have an acute condition within the abdomen requiring surgery. Some patients have had more than ten laparotomies. The pathophysiologic disturbance is felt to be an autonomic neuropathy. Patients may also have a peripheral neuropathy and hypothalamic dysfunction with inappropriate antidiuretic hormone (ADH) secretion and secondary hyponatremia.

The diagnosis can be made only by the demonstration in the urine of increased PBG. This can be done qualitatively by the Watson-Schwartz test or quantitatively by the use of chromatographic analysis.

Treatment is aimed at preventing acute attacks by avoiding as much as possible the known precipitating factors.

The overactivity of ALA synthetase may be caused by faulty feedback inhibition of the enzyme. This enzyme can be blocked experimentally by feeding a high carbohydrate diet. In some patients carbohydrate utilization may be impaired during the acute attacks, and insulin administration enhances the benefit of the high carbohydrate diet. These

Table 1-1. Reduction of excessive enzyme activity in acute intermittent porphyria

Biochemical defect	Liver ALA synthetase increased with urinary excretion of large amounts of delta ALA and PBG
Clinical signs	Abdominal pain; neurologic manifestations, including peripheral and autonomic nervous system dysfunction; many patients have hypertension; neurotic and psychotic behavior common
Diagnosis	Increased PBG in the urine; Watson-Schwartz test or chromatographic analysis
Treatment	Avoid known precipitating factors that may influence enzyme activity

AIP is the only inherited disturbance of porphyrin metabolism not associated with cutaneous sensitivity.

patients should avoid fasting. Low carbohydrate intake increases symptoms. AIP may represent a disease that we attempt to treat by the reduction of excessive enzyme activity (Table 1-1).

Pyridoxine deficiency, produced by the administration of pyridoxine analog, lowers ALA and PBG excretion in AIP. Pyridoxyl phosphate is a PBG cofactor for ALA synthetase. Since pyridoxine derivatives are required as cofactors for many other enzyme reactions, vitamin B_6 deficiency is not recommended as a form of therapy.

LIPID METABOLISM

Hereditary ataxic polyneuritis (Refsum's disease)

Forty-five cases of this disorder were described up to 1968. The disease is characterized by accumulation of phytanic acid, a branch chain fatty acid derived entirely from exogenous sources. It has been found in high concentration in these patients in the serum, liver, kidney, adipose tissue, and brain. The chemical block involves a failure of alpha oxidation of phytanic acid. It is transmitted as an autosomal recessive trait.

The relationship of the phytanic acid levels to clinical manifestations is unclear. High levels inhibit the oxidation of other fatty acids and may therefore interfere with brain metabolism. On the other hand, phytanic acid itself may have nothing to do with the clinical signs, but rather the enzyme that is deficient may be needed for oxidation of endogenous brain lipids as well as for phytanic acid. Support for this hypothesis of elevated serum phytanic acid in the asymptomatic mothers of two patients with the disease has been reported by Eldjarn and associates.[1, 2] As heterozygotes, they might have a sufficient amount of enzyme for normal neurologic function but an insufficient amount to metabolize large amounts of phytanic acid (Table 1-2).

In two patients reduction in serum phytanic acid was accomplished

Table 1-2. Hereditary ataxic polyneuritis (Refsum's disease)

Phytanic acid	Accumulation
Source	Exogenous
Block	Failure of α oxidation of phytanic acid Failure of oxidation of endogenous brain lipids (?)
Diagnosis	Detection of enzyme deficiency in fibroblasts

Table 1-3. Reduction of substrate or precursors in Refsum's disease

Clinical signs	Atypical retinitis pigmentosa Cerebellar ataxia Peripheral polyneuropathy Occasionally cataracts—usually posterior cortical Rarely corneal changes
Treatment	Reduction of serum phytanic acid Dietary restriction of chlorophyll and lipids

by omitting dietary sources of chlorophyll, of which phytanic acid is a major component, and by severely limiting lipids. There was little clinical improvement in these patients. To determine whether phytanic acid is toxic, it would be helpful to start treatment before clinical signs develop. The enzymatic defect can be detected in fibroblast cultures so that the diagnosis of the asymptomatic patient is now possible (Table 1-3).[3]

Cerebral lipidoses

Remarkable progress has been achieved in the past few years toward the elucidation of the biochemical abnormalities in inheritable lipid storage diseases. Patients with these diseases present a wide variety of medical problems confronting internists, neurologists, hematologists, orthopedic surgeons, general surgeons, radiologists, dermatologists, geneticists, pathologists, clinical chemists, as well as ophthalmologists. Abnormalities of lipid metabolism should always be suspected in infants whose mental development is slower than normal, especially if there is concomitant splenomegaly and hepatomegaly. There is a particular class of lipids, designated as sphingolipids, that characteristically are constructed from a common backbone called ceramide. This component consists of the N-acyl derivative of sphingosine in which a long-chain fatty acid is linked by an amide bond. Various substitutes are attached to carbon atom 1 of the sphingosine moiety of ceramide (Table 1-4).

In all the lipidoses in which the metabolic defect has been conclusively identified, the lesion has been demonstrated to be a deficiency of a specific catabolic enzyme. The highest activity of sphingolipid

Table 1-4. Enzymatic defects in sphingolipidoses

Disease	*Enzyme involved*
Gaucher's	Glucocerebrosidase
Metachromatic leukodystrophy	Sulfatidase (aryl sulfatase A)
Niemann-Pick	Sphingomyelinase
Fabry's	Ceramide trihexosidase
Generalized gangliosidosis	B-galactosidase
Tay-Sachs	B-N-acetyl hexosaminidase

hydrolyses is found in the subcellular particles called lysosomes. These observations strongly suggest that the sphingolipidoses belong to the group of lysosomal diseases. Our understanding of the nature of the metabolic defects in lipid storage diseases improved substantially during the past 5 years. The enzymatic lesions in Gaucher's disease, metachromatic leukodystrophy, Niemann-Pick, Fabry's disease, and generalized gangliosidosis are now established convincingly. Preliminary evidence of the metabolic defect in globoid leukodystrophy requires confirmation. The enzymatic lesion in Tay-Sachs disease has recently been disclosed with the use of labeled Tay-Sachs ganglioside.

However, it is conceivable that the metabolic derangement in Tay-Sachs disease is not strictly analogous to the deficiencies of catabolic enzymes in other lipid storage diseases. Perhaps in Tay-Sachs disease we are dealing with the accumulation of a fragment of membrane or membrane components that are not metabolized or even reassembled from individual components in situ. Information regarding the metabolism of membranes is extremely scanty at the present time. We may therefore be compelled to undertake extensive investigations along these lines in order to unravel the mystery of Tay-Sachs disease.

Metabolism of sphingolipids touches many other aspects of medicine in addition to the lipidoses. In studies of atherosclerosis, for example, the percentage increase of sphingomyelin in arteriosclerotic aortas is nearly the same order of magnitude as that of cholesterol. The significance of this finding is still unknown, although it has been confirmed in many laboratories.

It is possible that information regarding the factors that control galactocerebroside and sphingomyelin metabolism may enhance our comprehension of events that occur in patients with multiple sclerosis. There is also some evidence that the ganglioside composition of cells may be transformed in certain malignancies.

Gaucher's disease

Patients with Gaucher's disease, in which there is an accumulation of glucocerebrosides, have been divided into three clinical forms designated as infantile, juvenile, and adult. The infantile form has pronounced involvement of the central nervous system, while there is virtual absence of neural dysfunction in patients with the juvenile and adult types. Patients with the infantile form fail to exhibit normal mental development. Certain clinical aspects are shared by all three forms, such as splenomegaly, hepatomegaly, and erosion of the cortices of long bones and hip joints wth attendant pathologic features. The rate of progression of these features is much more rapid in the infantile and juvenile forms than in the adult type. Hemorrhagic tendencies may occur in these patients because of thromobocytopenia as well as mild anemia and leukopenia. Hematologic abnormalities usually respond favorably to splenectomy. Gaucher cells, in which there is a remarkable reticular pattern in the cytoplasm, are seen in bone marrow aspirates. These cells do not stain positive for fat with oil Red O or other lipid stains but strongly stain for carbohydrates with Schiff's periodic acid and Fuchsin's reagent. Similar staining cells may be found in histologic sections of the spleen, liver, and brain of patients with the infantile form of Gaucher's disease. These staining characteristics are in accord with the generally accepted assumption that the cells are filled with cerebroside.

Genetics

Gaucher's disease is generally considered to be a consequence of an inherited autosomal recessive defect, but a few instances of possible dominant genetic transmission have been reported. There are marked symptomalogic differences in patients with various forms of Gaucher's disease, and there are various rates of progression of the disease. Because of this, it is likely that the disease is a genetically heterogenous condition.

Biochemical lesion

The accumulation of glucocerebroside in various tissues of patients with Gaucher's disease has been established. Identification of cerebroside led to speculation over an abnormality of carbohydrate metabolism in Gaucher's disease. This was later excluded by chemical studies that ruled out the possibility of overproduction of a normal, although minor, tissue constituent. Although the final possibility of a deficiency of a catabolic enzyme was most difficult to demonstrate, it has eventually been shown to be responsible. An enzyme that catalyzed a hydrolytic cleavage of the glucose moiety of glucocerebroside was demonstrated in many human tissues. The enzyme was most active in the spleen; it was partially purified, and its properties were investigated. The activity of glucocerebrosidase in a series of 38 patients with the adult form of Gaucher's disease was 15% of that in the controls. Glucocerebrosidase activity was nearly completely absent in tissues of patients with the infantile form of Gaucher's disease. Extracts of normal human brain tissue also exhibit glucocerebrosidase activity, and this activity was also very low in preparations from patients with the infantile form of Gaucher's disease.

Most of the glucocerebroside found in peripheral tissue of patients with Gaucher's disease apparently originates from senescent leukocytes. The principal glycolipid of polymorphonuclear leukocytes is ceramide lactoside. Nearly 400 mg. of this substance must be catabolized as a consequence of the turnover of white blood cells. This metabolic feature becomes especially significant in patients with chronic myelogous leukemia, since characteristic lipid-laden Gaucher cells are frequently found in the bone marrow and spleen of such patients. However, only small quantities of glucocerebroside accumulate in the spleen of patients with chronic myelogenous leukemia. This accumulation probably reflects an overwhelming influx of glycolipids from myeloid cells. Glucocerebrosidase activity in the spleen increases when augmented quantities of glycolipid precursors are presented to the spleen for catabolism. Apparently, some patients with chronic myelogenous leukemia cannot effect a sufficient increase in the total activity of this enzyme to hydrolyze all of the glucocerebroside that arises in this condition. Glucocerebroside may also arise from glycolipid components of the erythrocyte membrane. A daily quantity of glucocerebroside that arises from erythocytorrhexis is probably 1/40 to 1/20 of that from the ceramide lactoside of leukocytes.

The glucocerebroside that accumulates in neuronal cells in some patients with the infantile form of Gaucher's disease probably arises from substances called gangliosides. The turnover of gangliosides is rather active in the early neonatal period and diminishes greatly as one matures. Patients with the adult form of Gaucher's disease apparently possess sufficient, although attenuated, glucocerebrosidase activity to dispose of the glucocerebroside that arises during the period of rapid ganglioside catabolism. They therefore escape mental difficulties from intraneuronally accumulated glucocerebroside (Table 1-5).

Diagnosis

The diagnosis of Gaucher's disease can generally be made with confidence by the presence of splenomegaly, hepatomegaly, bone involvement, and the finding of Gaucher cells in the bone marrow. There is a greatly increased plasma acid phosphatase activity. The amount of glucocerebroside in tissues obtained by biopsy can be determined by analytical methods. One can measure the glucocerebrosidase activity in washed leukocytes in a small sample of venous blood. A differential determination of white cells should be performed when this test is used, since the enzyme is primarily found in the polymorphonuclear leukocytes. A complete hematologic evaluation is especially important, since an

Table 1-5. Gaucher's disease

Enzymatic defect	Glucocerebroside + H_2O $\xrightarrow{\text{glucocerebrosidase}}$ Glucose + Ceramide
Forms	Infantile (fatal), juvenile, adult (chronic)
Genetics	Autosomal recessive (adult) (?) irregular dominant mode (infantile) (?)
Biochemical defect	Accumulation of glucocerebroside;deficiency of glucocerebrosidase
Ophthalmologic signs	Strabismus, paralytic; pingueculae—yellow-brown wedge-shaped, bilaterally present in 25% of the patients; perimacular degenerative changes
Other clinical signs	Hepatosplenomegaly, lymphadenopathy; erosion of the cortices of long bones with pathologic fractures; infantile form—severe neurologic disorders; adult form—hypersplenism and abnormal skin pigmentation

increase in the activity of glucocerebrosidase is seen in leukocyte preparations of patients with myelogenous leukemia and because hypersplenism is often present in Gaucher's disease.

A deficiency of glucocerebrosidase is also seen in fibroblasts in skin biopsies obtained from patients with Gaucher's disease and grown in tissue culture. Particularly interesting results were obtained in tissue culture of the skin fibroblasts from a family consisting of the parents, a sibling, and a child, the propositus, with the infantile form of Gaucher's disease. The activity of the glucocerebrosidase in tissue culture from the propositus was 3% of the control level. The activity of this enzyme in the cultures from the father and mother and unaffected sibling was 64%, 53%, and 44% of that found in a series of normal controls. If these observations can be confirmed by additional studies of families of patient with Gaucher's disease, it could provide a method for detecting heterozygous carriers with the Gaucher trait. Such a procedure would be extremely desirable because of the opportunity afforded for accurate genetic counseling.

Glucocerebrosidase activity has also been found in good titer in tissue cultures of fetal cells obtained by amniocentesis. A competent obstetrician can obtain a sufficient supply of these cells for tissue culture without danger of fetal or maternal harm during the fourth month of pregnancy. Approximately 5 weeks are required for the growth of enough cells for enzymatic assay. Thus, amniocentesis enables the physician to make the antenatal diagnosis of Gaucher's disease (Table 1-6).

Treatment

Homogenous preparations of human and beef spleen glucocerebrosidases have recently been prepared. Thus, the therapeutic attempts involving the exogenous administration of purified glucocerebrosidase ap-

Table 1-6. Gaucher's disease—diagnosis and treatment

Diagnosis	Splenomegaly, hepatomegaly, bone involvement
	Gaucher's cells in bone marrow
	Serum acid phosphatase elevated
	Tissue concentration of glucocerebroside elevated
	Glucocerebrosidase activity (washed leukocytes) decreased (to exclude myelogenous leukemia in which glucocerebrosidase activity is increased)
	Glucocerebrosidase activity decreased in fibroblasts (family analysis)
	Glucocerebrosidase activity decreased in fetal cells—amniocentesis
Treatment	Glucocerebrosidase (human, beef) replacement
	Splenectomy—hemorrhagic abnormalities
	Enzyme—amino acid arrangement (?)
	RNA messenger, DNA code—to correct enzyme synthesis (?)
	Splenic transplants (?)
	(Expose patient's cells to correct DNA cistran in tissue culture; reimplantation into host)

pear to be an imminent possibility. The most likely candidates for attempts at enzyme replacement would probably be patients who exhibit very low tissue levels of glucocerebrosidase activity, who are clinically rapidly deteriorating and who have hepatomegaly, splenomegaly, and bone marrow involvement. There is considerable evidence to indicate that exogenously administered enzymes are taken up by reticuloendothelial cells, which is precisely what is desired in patients with lipid storage disease. There is indication that exogenous enzymes can effectively reduce the intracellular accumulation of certain substances in intact cells. Patients with slow progression of the adult form of Gaucher's disease probably have approached a clinically stable condition by compensatory hepatomegaly and splenomegaly. Except for the hematologic abnormalities that may require splenectomy, it seems unnecessary to resort to novel therapeutic trials in these patients.

The isolation of glucocerebrosidase in a pure state now permits consideration of other possible forms of therapy. Is the synthesis of the enzyme repressed or does it proceed at normal or even increased rate in patients with Gaucher's disease? Is there an alteration in the amino acid sequence of the enzyme in patients with Gaucher's disease? There are methods for fingerprinting the peptide in the structure of proteins. It is possible that there is a multiplicity of enzyme alterations in patients with Gaucher's disease because they show so many variable ranges of enzyme activities. Perhaps a single alteration could be found in various afflicted members of one family. Perhaps it would be possible to extrapolate back to the base sequence of the messenger RNA and eventually to the DNA code for the enzyme. If so, then consideration could be given to the administration of substances of this type, with the hope that the synthesis of new correct enzymes would be directed to occur under these circumstances.

There is also the possibility of organ replacement in patients with very severe deficiency of glucocerebrosidases. A degree of success with splenic transplants has been cited in recent reports. We may look for further improvement in this area. This type of therapy might prove useful for patients with the infantile form of Gaucher's disease in which it seems unlikely that exogenously administered enzyme or polynucleotide type messengers would penetrate the blood brain barrier. Finally, it may be possible to alter the enzyme content for more production of the patient's own cells by exposing them to correct DNA cistran in tissue culture, followed by their reimplantation in the original host. Such a procedure would seem less likely to cause untoward effects than procedures involving organ or homologous enzyme replacement. When one attempts to establish enzyme production in deficient cells by metabolic cooperativity or by hydridization of cells, he must be cautious, since spontaneous malignant transformation of cells in tissue cultures is a well-recognized and not infrequent phenomenon if repeated passages are made. Also, rejection of the implanted cells by the host is a possibility (Table 1-6).

Niemann-Pick disease

The majority of patients with Niemann-Pick (N-P) disease are infants with severe mental retardation, cachexia, and hepatomegaly. The bone marrow may be involved but usually not so extensively as in patients with the infantile form of Gaucher's disease. There may be a moderate degree of splenomegaly. Appearance of a cherry red spot in the macular area has been reported in about one-third of these children. Some show an olive brown discoloration of their skin; a large, waxy, birefringent lipid-laden cell is seen in bone marrow smears, a cell that is probably derived from the reticuloendothelial system and that stains for both lipid and phosphorous.

Biochemical lesion

The lipid that accumulates in various tissues of the patient with N-P disease is sphingomyelin. It is a normal component of myelin and is a major lipid constituent of the plasma membrane, mitochondria, and microsomes in all mammalian cells. Studies of the biosynthesis of sphingomyelin in patients with N-P disease show no increase in the rate of sphingomyelin biosynthesis. This observation suggests that the metabolic defect in this condition is a deficiency of a catabolic enzyme. This hypothesis has been shown to be correct. The first step in the metabolism of sphingomyelin is the hydrolytic cleavage of the phosphorylcholine portion of the molecule.

Table 1-7. Niemann-Pick disease

Form	Infantile type A, B, C, and possibly D
Ocular sign	Cherry red spot in macular area
Other clinical signs	Hepatosplenomegaly, mental retardation, cachexia, and pulmonary involvement
Biochemical defect	Deficiency of catabolic enzyme—sphingomyelinase

$$\text{Sphingomyelin} + H_2O \xrightarrow{\text{Sphingomyelinase}} \text{Phosphorylcholine and ceramide}$$

Hepatic tissue is the most active source of this enzyme. A very drastic reduction in the level of sphingomyelinase activity was found in liver and subsequently in other tissues in patients with N-P disease. It was concluded that this is the primary metabolic defect in the disease. The rate of sphingomyelin accumulation allows one to divide N-P disease into types A, B, C, and possibly D. Less sphingomyelinase is present in the rapidly progressive disease. There is also a concomitant, although lesser, accumulation of cholesterol with sphingomyelin in tissues of patients with N-P disease. There is a variant of this disease labeled type D, a so-called Nova Scotia variant, in which no deficiency of sphingomyelinase can be demonstrated. In this latter type there is a preponderant accumulation of cholesterol in tissues in comparison to the amount of sphingomyelin. Perhaps in this group there is a possibility that the primary metabolic abnormality is an accumulation of cholesterol plus a moderate ancillary storage of sphingomyelin (Table 1-7).

Diagnosis

The diagnosis of N-P disease must always be considered in retarded infants with organomegaly and foam cells in their bone marrow. Diagnosis can be established by direct quantitative analysis of the concentration of sphingomyelin in biopsy specimens of the liver or by determination of sphingomyelinase activity in sonicated leukocyte preparations. The test is reliable and is rather easily carried out with radioactive sphingomyelinase substrate.

Deficiency of sphingomyelinase activity in patients with N-P disease is also actively reflected in enzyme assays performed on extracts of fibroblasts grown in tissue culture from biopsies of skin and bone marrow. The classical infantile form of N-P disease type A shows 3% of the control level of sphingomyelinase. About 10% of the control level is found in patients with N-P disease type B a more slowly progressive form than type A. It is possible that assays of sphingomelinase activity in tissue cultures of skin fibroblasts will prove to be a useful method for detect-

Table 1-8. Niemann-Pick disease—diagnosis

Mental retardation
Organomegaly
Foam cells in bone marrow
Sphingomyelin in liver biopsy
Sphingomyelinase activity decreased in leukocytes
Sphingomyelinase activity decreased in fibroblasts
N-P type A—3% of control activity
N-P type B—10% of control activity
Sphingomyelinase activity decreased in fetal cells obtained by amniocentesis

ing heterozygous carriers of N-P disease. It also seems probable that sphingomyelinase assays performed on tissue culture of fetal cells obtained by amniocentesis will permit the antenatal diagnosis of N-P disease (Table 1-8).

Treatment

Most of the concepts considered for the treatment of Gaucher's disease are generally applicable to treatment of patients with N-P disease. A highly active preparation for sphingomyelinase has been obtained from *Clostridium perfringens.* It is not known whether such a bacterial enzyme preparation would be tolerated by human patients in trials of enzyme replacement. A word of caution is required: since sphingomyelin is such a ubiquitous component of membranes, the parenteral administration of a highly active sphingomyelinase preparation may be potentially hazardous.

Tay-Sachs disease

Afflicted children from ethnic groups other than the Ashkenazic Jewish heritage are only rarely encountered. Infants with Tay-Sachs disease show severe progressive mental retardation and eventual blindness. The disease becomes manifest at about 5 months of age, and the patients generally die at about 2 years of age. A cherry red spot is seen in the macula in the majority of these infants. There is relatively little organomegaly or skeletal deformity except for the head, which is about 40% larger than normal.

Histologic examination of the brain reveals the presence of swollen neurons with concentrically layered cytoplasmic inclusion bodies. These densely staining bodies are comprised of cholesterol, phospholipids, and ganglioside. About 20% of the dry weight of these cytoplasmic bodies is protein. Except for the disproportionate increase in ganglioside, these substances are exactly the materials of which cell membranes are comprised.

The ganglioside that accumulates in neurons and to a lesser extent

Table 1-9. Tay-Sachs disease—chemistry of pathologic conditions

Swollen neurons	cytoplasmic inclusion bodies ↓ cholesterol, phospholides, ganglioside ↓ 20% protein—dry weight
Ganglioside	Monosialoceramide trihexoside (Tay-Sachs ganglioside)
Major brain gangliosides (Tay-Sachs ganglioside) terminal galactose absent	
Deficiency of galactose transferring enzyme—No	
B-N-Acetylgalactosaminidase—2 isoenzymes normally, deficiency of one in Tay-Sachs	

Table 1-10. Tay-Sachs disease

Genetics	Autosomal recessive
Frequency	1 in 10,000 births of Ashkenazic Jewish parentage
Carriers	1 in 50 of this group
Diagnosis	Clinical characteristics: onset at 5 months of age, fatal at 2 years of age, cherry red spot in the macula; enlarged head
	Preclinical characteristics: deficiency of hexosaminidase-A in leukocytes, fibroblasts
Therapy	Therapeutic abortion (?)

in peripheral tissues of patients with Tay-Sachs disease is a monosialoceramide trihexoside that is also called Tay-Sachs ganglioside. This compound differs from the major brain gangliosides by the absence of the terminal moiety of galactose. This suggests that there is a deficiency of a galactose transferring enzyme required for the biosynthetic completion of ganglioside. There is no evidence for this at the present time.

Other enzymes have been sought. The most recent development in this area is a finding by Okada and O'Brien[4, 5] that most tissues contain two enzymes or isoenzymes that catalyze the hydrolysis of beta-N-acetyl galactosaminide. These enzymes can be distinguished from each other by starch gel electrophoresis. Okada and O'Brien believe that one of these components is missing in tissues of patients with Tay-Sachs disease. This has been confirmed by others. Brady,[6] for example, feels that there is a deficiency of a specific hexosaminidase in patients with Tay-Sachs disease, which is normally required for the enzymatic hydrolysis of the N acetyl galactosaminide moiety of Tay-Sachs ganglioside (Table 1-9).

No special diagnostic skills are required for patients with Tay-Sachs disease because of its striking clinical characteristics. However, it may be possible to detect the presence of this condition before clinical manifestations become apparent. Okada and O'Brien believe that these patients have an absence of hexosaminidase-A in leukocytes and skin fibroblasts

Table 1-11. Fabry's disease

Enzyme deficiency	Ceramide trihexosidase with accumulation of ceramide trihexoside and dihexoside
Signs	
Ocular	Cataract, retinal edema, corneal opacities
Skin	Angiokeratoma
Genetic	Sex-linked
Treatment	Renal dialysis (transplant? enzyme replacement?)

grown in tissue culture. If this finding can be confirmed, it should prove a facile procedure for the early detection of patients at risk and perhaps for the antenatal diagnosis of Tay-Sachs disease.

There is no specific therapy except possible therapeutic abortion if the antenatal diagnosis can be made (Table 1-10).

Fabry's disease

Fabry's disease is a metabolic disorder, with sex-linked inheritance, in which the glycolipids and ceramide trihexoside and dihexoside accumulate. Fabry's disease is also called glycolipid lipidosis. The enzyme deficiency is postulated to be ceramide trihexosidase.

The clinical features result from the alterations produced by deposits of lipids. Usually the skin involvement is the earliest manifestation of the disease. The skin lesions are dilated, blood-filled capillaries in the upper dermis that often elevate the epidermis. The lesions do not blanch with pressure and are densest from the knees to the umbilicus. They are called angiokeratoma. Other clinical signs include episodic bouts of fever and painful extremities. Renal involvement with proteinuria and eventual renal failure is a common clinical course. Hypertensive cardiovascular and cerebrovascular disease are also common clinical findings. Death is usually from uremia or vascular disease, and most patients die between 40 and 50 years of age.

Ocular findings include involvement of the conjunctiva, cornea, or retina. There may be tortuosity of the retinal and conjunctival vessels, with retinal edema. There may be corneal epithelial opacities, which are probably secondary to lipid deposition. Lens opacities may also be present.

Diagnosis in males is usually made possible clinically from the history and from the findings of the characteristic skin rash and corneal dystrophy. Skin and renal biopsies may aid in the diagnosis. A complete ophthalmologic evaluation may help to confirm the diagnosis if corneal epithelium involvement is found and if there are dilated retinal veins.

There is no specific effective therapy available at this time. Most treatment is aimed at the management of the renal and cardiovascular complications and the symptomatic relief of pain (Table 1-11).

Lesch-Nyhan syndrome

The Lesch-Nyhan syndrome was first described in 1963. The full clinical picture consists of mental retardation, choreoathetosis, spastic cerebral palsy, self-mutilation, and aggressive behavior associated with hyperuricemia and possible tophaceous gout in later life. It is transmitted as an X-linked recessive characteristic and occurs only in young males.

Urate synthesis is increased about 20 times, with greatly increased urinary excretion of uric acid. Seegmiller[7, 8] in 1967 demonstrated that erythrocytes and skin fibroblasts lack the enzyme hypoxanthine guanine phosphoribosyl transferase (HGPRT). This enzyme normally converts hypoxanthine and guanine in the presence of phosphoribosyl-pyrophosphate back to inosinic and guanylic acid.

However, Marks and associates[9] in 1968 detected a child with Lesch-Nyhan syndrome at 94 hours of age and treated him with allopurinol (a xanthine oxidase inhibitor); the serum uric acid level became normal. This treatment did not prevent the development of mental retardation, spasticity, and self-mutilation. Also complicating the picture are patients with the clinical syndrome, including hyperuricemia, but normal levels of HGPRT.

An incomplete deficiency of HGPRT causes a reduced but still excessive purine synthesis that clinically presents in late adolescence or early adulthood with gouty arthritis and a mild neurologic deficit.

Children who are affected with a complete deficiency usually appear normal at birth, but by 4 months of age there is some neurologic dysfunction. The characteristic choreoathetosis and spasticity develop within the first year or two of life.

Gouty arthritis is usually not a major problem despite the marked overproduction of uric acid; but gouty nephropathy, or uric acid renal calculi, or both, with secondary renal dysfunction is a common and serious complication. The early diagnosis of children affected with this disorder is important because the renal dysfunction caused by the hyperuricemia can be managed with allopurinol. The neurologic dysfunction does not respond to this therapy.

However, some children with complete HGPRT deficiency may not have elevated blood uric acid levels, but all children excrete excessive quantities of uric acid in the urine. However, other conditions, such as leukemia, also can cause increased urinary excretion of uric acid, and a blood sample should be assayed for the HGPRT enzyme.

Since treatment at the present is ineffective, in utero diagnosis and therapeutic abortion for confirmed cases appears to offer the best control of the disease (Table 1-12).

Table 1-12. Lesch-Nyhan syndrome

Pathogenesis	Unclear
Deficiency	Hypoxanthine guanine phosphoribosyl transferase (HGPRT) enzyme
Increase	Purine synthesis
Signs	Self-mutilation, choreoathetosis, mental retardation, and spasticity
Diagnosis	Hyperuricemia
	Xanthine, hypoxanthine, and uric acid increased in blood, urine, and amniotic fluid
	Blood assay of HGPRT activity
Therapy	Allopurinol reduces uric acid, but symptoms persist
	Purine synthesis inhibition (adenine and 6-methyl mercaptopurine); symptoms persist

AMINO ACID METABOLISM

Phenylketonuria

In 1934 Folling[10] described ten patients, several of them sibs, who excreted phenylpyruvic acid in the urine and were mentally deficient. Jervis[11] demonstrated the inheritance to be of autosomal recessive transmission. It was shown that the metabolic defect was in the conversion of phenylalanine to tyrosine, with the subsequent accumulation of phenylalanine. In 1953 Jervis reported that the enzyme phenylalanine hydroxylase in the liver was inactive.

Clinically, the disease manifests itself by the elevation of plasma phenylalanine to 30 times the normal level and by the excretion of phenylpyruvic acid in the urine. Usually, by 6 months of age there is some evidence of retarded mental development. Other signs are eczema, seizures, reduced pigmentation of the hair and skin, blue eyes and blond hair, and hyperreflexia. EEG abnormalities in 80% of the patients with phenylketonuria; microcephaly in 68%; hyperactive reflexes in 63%; eczema in 19% to 34%, depending on the clinical series; and seizures in 26% have been reported; 35% of these patients could not walk, and 62% could not talk.

Examination of pathologic specimens has shown widespread deficient myelinization, with secondary gliosis and associated microcephaly. The chemical basis for this is not fully understood. The pathologic findings account, however, for many of the neurologic symptoms.

The primary treatment modality is to reduce phenylalanine intake to that which is necessary for the growth and repair of tissues and to prevent its accumulation. A casein hydrolysate with phenylalanine removed by treatment with charcoal has been prepared. All the biochemical abnormalities of phenylketonuria can be reversed by a low phenylalanine diet, but one must be very careful to ensure adequate dietary intake to maintain growth because hypophenylalaninemia may, in itself, impair development of the nervous system. Also, clinical improvement of the eczema and of the hair and skin pigmentation occurs during dietary treatment. Many of the neurologic findings also improve with treatment. It has been shown that the low phenylalanine diet in patients can reverse recent intellectual impairment.

Mabry[11a] demonstrated that it is very important to treat pregnant women who have phenylketonuria with an appropriate dietary regimen in order to protect the fetus from hyperphenylalaninemia. The placenta does not protect the child, even if he eventually is documented to be a heterozygote, and he will be retarded from the in utero exposure to hyperphenylalaninemia. In 25 pregnancies of untreated phenylketonuric mothers, Mabry reported that all offspring were retarded, with I.Q.'s equal to or lower than that of the mother. None of these 25 children were homozygous.

The deficiency of the enzyme phenylalanine hydroxylase, with the subsequent accumulation of phenylalanine, causes many other secondary biochemical changes, all of which appear to be indirectly related to the accumulation of phenylalanine and its chemical derivatives. Tyrosine metabolism is altered, and there is a suggestion that catecholamine synthesis may also be impaired. The pigment dilution is caused by impaired melanin synthesis.

Testing a newborn's blood for phenylalanine has become a legal requirement in many states and is carried out about the third day of life. Values above 6 mg. of phenylalanine per 100 ml. of plasma are highly suggestive of the disease. Diagnosis should be confirmed by repeated quantitative determination of the plasma for phenylalanine. In typical phenylketonuric patients, plasma phenylalanine values rise rapidly within the first 10 days of life to levels above 30 mg./100 ml.

With the mass screening programs that are now in use and with the proper dietary therapy, a patient with the clinical findings of phenylketonuria will hopefully become a medical curiosity (Table 1-13).

Albinism

Another disorder of amino acid metabolism is albinism, which is characterized by a decrease or absence of melanin in the skin, hair, and eyes. The melanocytes in albinos lack the enzyme tyrosinase, which hydroxylates tyrosine to dihydroxyphenylalanine (dopa). Dopa in turn is eventually converted to melanin. The incidence of albinism is about 1:20,000 and is more common in dark races.

There are three major clinical variants of albinism: oculocutaneous, or complete, ocular, and cutaneous, or partial, albinism. In oculocutaneous albinism there is an absence of normal pigmentation in the skin and hair and a deficiency of pigment in the retinal pigment epithelium. The

Table 1-13. Phenylketonuria

Accumulation	Phenylalanine and its metabolites
Source	Exogenous
Block	Deficiency of phenylalanine hydroxylase ⟶ (defect of hydroxylation of phenylalanine to tyrosine)
	Phenylalanine —(Phenylalanine hydroxylase)⟶ Tyrosine → thyroxine, melanine, epinephrine, oxidation
Signs	Mental retardation, albinism, photophobia
Diagnosis	Blood assay for phenylalanine
Treatment	Reduction of phenylalanine intake
Casein hydrolysate (most of phenylalanine removed) substituted	
Infants with elevations of 6 to 20 mg./100 ml.—need not treat	
Infants with elevations of 20 mg./100 ml. +—treat, but check levels	
Pregnant women with PKU—attempt dietary therapy during pregnancy in order to protect the fetus from in utero hyperphenylalaninemia; placenta does not protect fetus	

irides are translucent. The choroidal and retinal vascular patterns are very prominent, and there is a hypoplastic to aplastic macula that is probably the chief cause of the defective vision. Other associated findings are photophobia, nystagmus, and an average vision of about 20/200. Large refractive errors are very common with myopia, more common than hyperopia. The hereditary pattern of oculocutaneous albinism or complete albinism is of autosomal recessive transmission.

In ocular albinism the eye findings are the same as in oculocutaneous albinism, but the skin pigmentation is within the normal range. The inheritance of this disease is sex-linked recessive transmission. In cutaneous, or partial, albinism, the lack of pigment is localized only to the skin and hair, with no ocular involvement. On the head there is usually a bilateral symmetrical white forelock that is triangular in shape. There are also areas of the body with normal pigment and other areas that are unpigmented. The heredity in this condition is of autosomal dominant transmission. Earlier theories about the pathophysiology of albinism maintained that the condition was caused by an absence of melanocytes, but in 1952 Becker[12] reported that amelanotic melanocytes were present in albino skin.

Radioautography with C^{14}-labeled tyrosine has been utilized to assay tyrosinase activity. In the skin and hair bulbs of people with oculocutaneous albinism no tyrosinase activity has been detected. Also, in albinos the melanocytes have been consistently tyrosinase negative.

There is no specific treatment for this condition. The ocular symptoms can be improved if the patient wears dark sunglasses or tinted

Table 1-14. Albinism

Types	Oculocutaneous, or complete Ocular Cutaneous, or partial
Defect	Tyrosine —tyrosinase→ dopa
Signs	General—absence of pigment in hair and skin Ocular—translucent irides, reduced pigmentation of pigment epithelium of the eye, hypoplastic-aplastic macula, nystagmus, photophobia, decreased vision, ametropia
Treatment	Reduce illumination and dazzling through optical means; usually not very successful in improving vision

contact lenses. Pinhole contact lenses have been used in the newborn in an attempt to reduce the intraocular dazzling from the increased illumination in the hope that the macular function might develop more normally, but this has not proved to be very successful (Table 1-14).

Homocystinuria

Homocystinuria is an inborn error of sulfur–amino acid metabolism and was first described in 1962. Over 100 patients with homocystinuria have been reported. In frequency of inborn errors it ranks second to phenylketonuria. Signs include lens dislocation, joint laxity, vascular thrombosis, malar flush, and sometimes mental retardation.

The enzyme defect appears to be in the activity of cystathionine synthetase, which converts homocysteine and serine to cystathionine. The activity of this enzyme is reduced or absent in the liver, brain and fibroblasts. As a consequence, homocystine, the oxidized derivative of homocysteine and its precursor methionine, accumulates in blood and urine. The product of the reaction, cystathionine, is reduced in homocystinuric brains. Since cysteine is formed from cystathionine, the requirements for exogenous cysteine are increased in homocystinuria.

The pathogenesis has been attributed to homocysteine excess and to folate, cystathionine, and cysteine deficiencies. Some believe that the clinical severity correlates with plasma homocysteine levels.

The mental defect may be related to serum folate concentrations. A folic acid derivative is needed to methylate homocysteine to methionine. Therefore, if the supply of folate is low, more homocysteine would accumulate. Conversely, because of high concentrations of homocysteine, folate might be utilized more rapidly than in normal subjects, making the requirement for folate greater in patients with homocystinuria than in normal subjects (see Table 1-15).

Table 1-15. Homocystinuria

Accumulation	Homocysteine, methionine
Source	Exogenous
Block	Cystathionine synthetase deficient (homocysteine and serine ⟶ cystathionine)
Pathogenesis	Excess—homocysteine Deficiencies—folate, cystathionine, and cysteine
Signs	Lens dislocation, vascular thrombosis as a cause of death, mental retardation, joint laxity, malar flush
Diagnosis	Homocysteine in blood and urine Amniotic fluid cells

Therapy

Restriction of dietary methionine lowers plasma methionine and homocystine levels. A special low methionine diet is available. Lentils, gelatine, and soya are protein sources low in methionine. A low methionine diet should be supplemented with cystine or cysteine. The addition of folate or choline, which facilitates the methylation of homocysteine to methionine also reduces homocysteine while further increasing blood methionine. It is not known if this increase in concentration of methionine is toxic in this disorder.

In some but not all patients with homocystinuria, pyridoxine doses of 150 to 1,200 mg. a day results in some reduction of blood homocysteine. Pyridoxine administration has been associated with the onset of seizures as well as with the termination of seizures. The mechanism of pyridoxine effectiveness is unclear. Although methionine restriction and folate and pyridoxine supplementation may reduce blood and urine homocystine, there is as yet no evidence that they have clinical benefit, particularly in older patients. No clinical change, other than an occasional improvement in behavior, has been reported.

Therapy has also been directed at increasing cystathionine concentrations. No report of clinical change as yet is available. The administration of cysteine alone has not resulted in clinical improvement.

The infusion of large amounts of arginine glutamate increases homocysteine secretion, presumably by competing with homocysteine for renal tubular reabsorption. Perhaps this could be helpful in treatment of acute vascular thrombosis. Virtually every therapeutic possibility seems to have been explored in homocystinuria. Until more is known about its pathogenesis or until a large number are treated in a similar manner from early life, little will be learned about the management of this disorder (Table 1-16).

Table 1-16. Reduction of substrates or its precursors—homocystinuria

Restrict methionine ⟶ reduced plasma methionine and homocysteine (lentils, soya, gelatin—low in methionine)
Supplement with cystine or cysteine
Add folate or choline—facilitates methylation of homocysteine ⟶ methionine
Pyridoxine 150 to 1,200 mg. per day—reduction of blood homocysteine complex of pyridoxal phosphate + homocysteine
Add cystathione
Arginine glutamate infusions—increases homocystine excretion
Value of therapy (?)

Table 1-17. Reduction of substrate or its precursors—galactosemia

Disaccharidase deficiencies	*Prevention and treatment*
Lactase	Avoid milk, pills, capsules, syrups
Sucrose	Avoid sucrose
Isomaltase	Add fungal sucrose
Galactokinase	Avoid galactose
Galactose-1-phosphate uridyl transferase	Avoid galactose
Fructose-1-phosphate aldolase	Avoid fructose

It should be stressed that it is possible to detect this disorder in the fetus by examination of amniotic fluid cells.

SUGAR METABOLISM

Galactosemia

Galactosemia is one of the disaccharidase deficiencies that are examples of disease entities in which it is necessary to reduce the amount of substrate or its precursors, since the host is unable to metabolize the substrate (Table 1-17).

Galactosemia is a congenital and hereditary disorder in the metabolism of galactose. There is an impairment in the utilization of ingested galactose and its conversion to glucose or energy. Galactosemia is usually caused by the absence of galactose-1-phosphate uridyl transferase, but an elevated blood and urine galactose level can be caused by the absence of galactokinase. The disease is transmitted as autosomal recessive.

Galactose-1-phosphate uridyl transferase converts galactose-1-phosphate to glucose-1-phosphate. Galactokinase converts galactose to galactose-1-phosphate, and the conversion requires adenosine triphosphate (ATP). Patients with the transferase deficiency have the full clinical picture, while patients with the kinase deficiency usually have only cataracts (Table 1-18). Accumulation of galactose-1-phosphate in transferase but not in kinase deficiency may cause a depletion of ATP, and

Table 1-18. Galactosemia

Accumulation	Galactose
Source	Exogenous
Block	Galactokinase
	Galactose-1-phosphate uridyl transferase
Clinical signs	Mental retardation
	Cataracts (galactokinase deficiency and transferase)—other signs only with transferase deficiency
	Accumulation of galactitol in lens
	Cirrhosis, hepatosplenomegaly, vomiting, diarrhea, weight loss, lack of energy
	Self-perception disturbances
Diagnosis	Prenatal examination of amniotic fluid cells
	Blood-urine concentrations—galactosuria, amino aciduria, and albuminuria
	Erythrocyte assay for galactose-1-phosphate uridyl transferase

the loss of so important a source of high energy phosphate may account for most of the signs. Cataracts are caused by the accumulation of galactitol in the lens tissues in both deficiencies.

Treatment

If significant milk ingestion persists in patients with galactosemia, death usually results. If, however, the diagnosis is made before the disease is too far advanced, all the symptoms and signs may regress if patients are given galactose-free diets.

Withdrawal of galactose from the diet is the treatment for both deficiencies. In patients with transferase deficiency it eliminates vomiting and diarrhea, and restores weight gain. Cirrhosis is halted and some liver damage is reversed, but if cataracts have developed, they do not always disappear. Some patients in whom transferase deficiency is demonstrated may develop normally even when no treatment is administered or when treatment is started after 1 year. Thus, considerable variation in the clinical manifestations of the transferase deficiency exists and might complicate the evaluation of treatment.

Self-perception disturbances (such as poor self-image, inadequacy, and anxiety) that were unrelated to cataracts are frequently encountered among those treated for galactosemia, and may be caused by chronic illness or parental concern about rigid exclusion of galactose from the diet rather than by galactosemia itself. Galactose-free formulas, such as Nutramigen, are available, and the composition of low galactose diets has been published. Lactose-containing milks, milk solids, drugs, and syrups are not tolerated. Peas, lima beans, sugar beets, liver, pancreas, and brain should be avoided. Meat base and soya bean formulas are low in galactose. There is no evidence that low galactose diets are harmful to infants. Galactose needed for brain lipid can be synthesized from glucose by the enzyme uridine diphosphate galactose-4-epimicrase.

It is important to realize that galactosemia can be diagnosed prenatally by examination of cultured amniotic fluid cells. This examination should be performed on mothers who are known to have galactosemia, and in view of the possibility of damage to the fetus in utero, the mother's lactic intake should be limited until the diagnosis can be ruled out. Ethanol inhibits the oxidation of galactose, and its intake by a woman carrying a galactosemic fetus should be avoided.

DIAGNOSIS OF HERITABLE METABOLIC DEFECTS BY AMNIOCENTESIS

One way in which the births of many children with fatal diseases of genetic origin or with neonatal defects might be prevented is to make the diagnosis in utero. If the diagnosis can be accurately made, the future parents will have the opportunity to prevent the birth by therapeutic abortion, and they and the state will be spared a tremendous emotional and financial ordeal. Today, through the use of amniocentesis, karyotyping (determining the cell's chromosomal pattern), and tissue-culture techniques, a physician has the technologic know-how to make in utero diagnoses of disabling and fatal diseases of genetic origin.

In 1956 Fuchs and Riis[13] were able to make a fetal sex determination from amniotic fluid cells. After the development of amniotic fluid tissue culture, it became possible to demonstrate the fetal karyotype, and at least 15 cases of mongolism have been diagnosed prenatally.[14]

Diagnostic amniocentesis, performed transabdominally, first achieved clinical importance in the management of pregnancies complicated by Rh blood incompatibility. At the present time, over 300 amniocenteses have been done specifically for prenatal genetic studies and high-risk pregnancies.

An example of a high-risk pregnancy is one that occurs in families in which there has previously been the birth of a child affected with an inheritable metabolic disease and in which it has been demonstrated that both parents were carriers. It is estimated that 1 in every 200 live births has a significant chromosomal abnormality. It is known that chromosomal abnormalities increase with maternal age. The incidence of trisomy 21 (mongolism) is 1 per 2,300 births in women under 20 years of age, 1 in 290 births in women from 35 to 39 years of age, 1 in 100 births in women from 40 to 45 years of age, and reaches 1 in 46 births in women of 45 years of age.[15] In terms of all chromosomal abnormalities, a pregnant woman between 40 and 44 has about a 1:40 chance of bearing a chromosomally abnormal child.[16] Thus, for pregnant women over 40, routine diagnostic amniocentesis should be considered.

Also, if either parent is a known translocation carrier, the high risk of bearing a chromosomally abnormal child makes amniocentesis seem advisable.

In the largest series of amniocentesis—162 cases reported by Nadler and Gerbie[17]—160 were successfully performed, with a repeat procedure required only in 7. Amniotic fluid cells were successfully cultured in 155 of these cases. The authors reported no fetal or maternal complications.

The cultured amniotic fluid cells can be karyotyped, and any chromosomal abnormalities can be determined. Also, in some inheritable metabolic diseases, through the use of autoradiographic methods and radioactive-labeled substances, the cultured amniotic fluid cells have been shown to be deficient in certain enzymes.

A set of identical twins with Lesch-Nyhan syndrome has been diagnosed in utero.[18] Radioactive hypoxanthine and autoradiographic methods were utilized to show the deficient hypoxanthine guanine phosphoribosyl transferase activity, with the affected cells failing to incorporate hypoxanthine and remaining unlabeled.

Other inherited disorders of metabolism in which amniocentesis may play a role in antenatal diagnosis include Niemann-Pick disease, Gaucher's disease, Tay-Sachs disease, Refsum's disease, and galactosemia.

It was demonstrated by Holtz[19] in 1964 that cultured fibroblasts from patients with Niemann-Pick disease accumulate almost two times the amount of sphingomyelin as control cells accumulate. He also showed that fibroblasts derived from the amnion of an infant subsequently diagnosed as having Niemann-Pick disease also accumulated sphingomyelin. Sphingomyelinase activity has been demonstrated in cultured amniotic fluid fibroblasts. Thus, it may now be possible to diagnose Niemann-Pick disease in utero by assaying for sphingomyelinase activity.

In Gaucher's disease there has been a deficiency of the enzyme glucocerebrosidase, which hydrolyzes glucocerebroside. Cultured skin fibroblasts can be shown to have glucocerebrosidase activity, and since amniotic fluid fibroblasts also contain glucocerebrosidase activity, the in utero diagnosis of Gaucher's disease is possible.

In Tay-Sachs disease there is an accumulation of Gm_2 ganglioside in the central nervous system because of the absence of hexosaminidase-A, which is involved in the catabolism of sphingolipids. A case of Tay-Sachs disease has been diagnosed by Schneck and associates[20] during the second trimester of pregnancy. They were able to demonstrate a nearly complete absence of hexosaminidase-A activity in the amniotic fluid and the cultured amniotic fluid cells. Subsequently, in the abortus they demonstrated the enzyme deficiency in the liver and brain.

In Refsum's disease the fatty acid phytanic acid accumulates. Since Herndon and associates[21] have shown that cultured amniotic cells have the ability to oxidize phytanic acid, the prenatal diagnosis of Refsum's disease has become a possibility.

Amniocentesis can be used to diagnose galactosemia in utero. It

Table 1-19. Diagnosis of heritable metabolic defects by amniocentesis

Disease	*Prenatal diagnosis*
Hereditary ataxic polyneuritis (Refsum's)	Possible
Porphyria	Potentially possible
Galactosemia	Made
Homocystinuria	Possible
Gaucher's	Possible
Niemann-Pick	Possible
Tay-Sachs	Made
Fabry's	Potentially possible
Lesch-Nyhan syndrome	Made
Phenylketonuria	Potentially possible
Albinism	Potentially possible

was done on a known maternal heterozygote who had previously given birth to a child with galactosemia. The cultured amniotic fluid cells contained no galactose-1-phosphate uridyl transferase activity.[22] This diagnosis was confirmed by the absence in the cord blood of this enzyme activity.

Amniocentesis is a relatively new technique with vast possibilities. When combined with the new developments in the tissue culturing of amniotic cells and autoradiographic techniques for assessement of enzyme activity, it will enable physicians to make in utero diagnosis of heritable conditions that are life-threatening and fatal (Table 1-19).

REFERENCES

1. Eldjarn, L., Try, K., and others: Dietary effects on serum-phythanic acid levels and on clinical manifestations in heredopathia atactica polyneuritiforms, Lancet **1**:691, 1966.
2. Eldjarn, L.: Hereditary ataxic polyneuritis: biochemical and dietary studies, Clin. Biochem. **1**:273, 1968.
3. Steinberg, D., Herndon, J. H., Jr., and others: Refsum's disease: nature of the enzyme defect, Science **156**:1740, 1967.
4. Okada, S., and O'Brien, J. S.: Tay-Sachs disease: generalized absence of a beta-D-N-acetylhexosaminidase compound, Science **165**:698, 1969.
5. Okada, S., and O'Brien, J. S.: Generalized gangliosidosis: beta-galactosidase deficiency, Science **160**:1002, 1968.
6. Brady, R. O.: Sphingolipid metabolism in neural tissues, Neurosciences Research **2**:301, 1969.
7. Seegmiller, J. E.: The clinical significance of hyperuricemia, Med. Ann. D. C. **36**:215, 1967.
8. Seegmiller, J. E.: Lesch-Nyhan syndrome: Management and treatment, Fed. Proc. **27**:1097, 1968.
9. Marks, J. F., Baum, J., and others: Lesch-Nyhan syndrome treated from the early neonatal period, Pediatrics **42**:357, 1968.
10. Følling, A.: Über Ausscheidung von Phenylbrenztraubensäure in den Harn als Stoffwechselanomalie in Verbindung mit Imbezillitat, Ztschr. Physiol. Chem. **227**:169, 1934.
11. Jervis, G. A.: Studies on phenylpyruvic oligophrenia: phenylpyruvic acid content of blood, Proc. Soc. Exp. Biol. Med. **81**:715, 1952.

11a. Mabry, C. C., Denniston, J. C., and others: Maternal phenylketonuria: a cause of mental retardation in children without the metabolic defect, New Eng. J. Med. **269**:1404, 1965.
12. Becker, S. W., Jr., Fitzpatrick, T. B., and Montgomery, H.: Human melanogenesis: cytology and histology of pigment cells (melanodendrocytes), A.M.A. Arch. Dermat. & Syph. **65**:511, 1952.
13. Fuchs, F., and Riis, P.: Antenatal sex determination, Nature **177**:330, 1956.
14. Milunsky, A., Littlefield, J., and others: Prenatal genetic diagnosis, as quoted in New Eng. J. Med. **283**:1370, 1970.
15. Collmann, R. D., and Stoller, A.: A survey of mongoloid births in Victoria, Australia, 1942-1957, Amer. J. Public Health **52**:813, 1962.
16. Carter, C., and MacCarthy, D.: Incidence of mongolism and its diagnosis in newborn, Brit. J. Social Med. **5**:83, 1951.
17. Nadler, H. L., and Gerbie, A. B.: Role of amniocentesis in the intrauterine detection of genetic disorders, New Eng. J. Med. **282**:596, 1970.
18. Santo, G., and Felix, J. S.: Lesch-Nyhan mutation: prenatal detection with amniotic fluid cells, Science **155**:1682, 1967.
19. Holtz, A. I., Uhlendorf, B. W., and Frederickson, D. S.: Persistence of a lipid defect in tissue cultures derived from patients with Niemann-Pick disease, Fed. Proc. **23**:128, 1964.
20. Schneck, L., Valenti, C., and others: Prenatal diagnosis of Tay-Sachs disease, Lancet **1**:582, 1970.
21. Herndon, J. H., Jr., Steinberg, D., and Uhlendorf, B. W.: Refsum's disease: defective oxidation of phytanic acid in tissue cultures derived from homozygotes and heterozygotes, New Eng. J. Med. **281**:1034, 1969.
22. Nadler, H. L.: Antenatal detection of hereditary disorders, Pediatrics **42**:912, 1968.

Chapter 2

Toxicity of strong miotics in children

Leonard Apt, M.D.

The purpose of this chapter is first, to comment on selected known untoward effects of the long-acting anticholinesterase agents as they relate to children and second, to discuss two toxic manifestations of the drugs, which previously have not been emphasized or, possibly, recognized.

For the most part the discussion will pertain to the use of isoflurophate (Floropryl, DFP) and echothiophate (Phospholine) iodide in children who have strabismus but no other ocular disease.

ADVERSE REACTIONS

Local and systemic manifestations of parasympathetic hyperactivity may result from the accumulation of endogenous acetylcholine in effector organs or nerve tissue if its hydrolysis has been prevented by cholinesterase-inhibiting agents such as isoflurophate and echothiophate.

In general, children tolerate the potent long-acting miotics better than adults do and have fewer serious toxic effects.

The local toxic reactions from isoflurophate and echothiophate encountered in children and adults are given in the list below.

Pain in eye, brow, head
Photophobia and burning sensation
Vision dim, blurred
Eyelid muscle twitching
Hyperemia of conjunctiva; thickening and obstruction of tear ducts
Allergic blepharoconjunctivitis
Superficial punctate keratitis

Iris cysts
Irreversible miosis
Iridocyclitis
Pupillary block and angle-closure glaucoma
Cataract
Retinal detachment

Many children will complain of pain in or around the eye during the first few days of therapy, but the symptoms usually are transient and are easily controlled with analgesics.

Though children may have conjunctival hyperemia when using the miotics, they do not get thickening of the conjunctiva with obstruction of the tear ducts, as sometimes described in adults.

Since isoflurophate is used more commonly in children than in adults, allergic blepharoconjunctivitis is more frequently seen in young patients. Some children are hypersensitive to the peanut oil vehicle or to the ointment base.

Children have a greater tendency to form so-called iris cysts than adults do, when using the strong miotics. Concomitant use of phenylephrine hydrochloride eyedrops has reduced this complication.

Roy and associates[1] recently reported irreversible miosis in a 6-month-old infant after the use of echothiophate. I, too, have seen this complication, and it has not been limited only to very young infants.

Acute iridocyclitis with posterior synechiae has been reported in adults, but it is rare in children.

I know of no report of retinal detachment occurring in a child after the use of isoflurophate or echothiophate; however, the complication has been reported in adults.

Pupillary block with angle-closure glaucoma after the use of a strong miotic is rare in children. Jones and Watson[2] reported one case that occurred in a 7-year-old child. The complication is more commonly seen in adults.

Lens opacities have been seen only rarely in children receiving isoflurophate or echothiophate. Many children who have strabismus and are taking these drugs have been examined, and nearly all results of the examinations have been normal. Harrison[3] reported transient anterior subcapsular opacities that developed in a 13-year-old girl receiving isoflurophate. Axelsson and Nyman[4] reported this complication that developed in a 19-year-old patient treated with isoflurophate and in a 6-year-old child receiving echothiophate. It appears that the lens opacities caused by the long-acting anticholinesterase drugs are transient in the young patient but may progress in the elderly patient even after the medication has been stopped.

Systemic toxicity is associated with lowered blood cholinesterase

Table 2-1. Systemic toxicity of isoflurophate (Floropryl) and echothiophate (Phosopholine) iodide

System	*Toxic manifestation*
Gastrointestinal	Cramps, nausea, vomiting, diarrhea, eructation, pyrosis
Respiratory	Bronchospasm, cough, wheezing, chest tightness, pulmonary edema, cyanosis
Cardiovascular	Bradycardia, cardiac arrest, pallor, increased blood pressure
Genitourinary	Frequent, involuntary micturition
Muscle (striated)	Weakness, twitching, cramps
Glands (nasal mucous membrane, bronchial, lacrimal, salivary, sweat)	Rhinorrhea, increased bronchial secretion, lacrimation, salivation, sweating
Central nervous	Anxiety, restlessness, emotional lability, confusion, poor coordination, insomnia, nightmares, tremors, ataxia, dysarthria, convulsions, coma, Cheyne-Stokes respiration, circulatory and respiratory center depression, hypotension

levels. No consistent relationship exists, however, between symptoms and blood level. Untoward systemic effects are much more likely to occur with echothiophate than with isoflurophate. The disparity in effects can be explained by the dissimilar absorption charcteristics of the two drugs. Echothiophate is prepared in an aqueous solution and can be readily absorbed into the general circulation by way of the mucosal surfaces of the conjunctiva, nasopharynx, or gastrointestinal tract. Isoflurophate, on the other hand, is prepared in an anhydrous peanut oil vehicle or an ointment base, so systemic absorption is minimal or does not occur. Also, isoflurophate hydrolyzes promptly in the presence of water. Moisture in the conjunctival sac or nasolacrimal drainage system may inactivate some or all of the ophthalmic solution.

Children tend to have a lower incidence of troublesome side effects from echothiophate treatment than adults do (Table 2-1). Complaints of problems such as anorexia, nausea, abdominal cramps, diarrhea, and sweating occur in less than 10% of pediatric patients. Even when they do occur they are milder and of shorter duration than those experienced by adults.

We should be cognizant of the potential danger of prolonged apnea and even occasional death in patients with low blood cholinesterase levels caused by echothiophate treatment if succinylcholine is given with general anesthesia. Normally, succinylcholine is a short-acting, depolarizing muscle relaxant that, like acetylcholine, requires cholinesterase for its breakdown. A deficiency of plasma pseudocholinesterase permits the drug to maintain endplate depolarization and to prevent repolarization. Thus, the neuromuscular block persists. If a muscle relaxant is needed for endotracheal intubation and the anesthesiologist is aware of the potential problem, he can substitute a nondepolarizing agent, such as d-tubocurarine or gallamine triethiodide, which does not require cholinesterase for breakdown.

At the Jules Stein Eye Institute we commonly use intranasal intubation, thus eliminating the need for neuromuscular blocking agents.

NEW OBSERVATIONS

During the past several years two toxic manifestations of echothiophate and isoflurophate therapy that deserve attention have been recognized by the author.

Hyperreactivity in Down's syndrome

The first adverse reaction is the remarkable hyperreactivity to echothiophate exhibited by several children with Down's syndrome (mongolism). The patients had almost identical histories. They were seen at approximately 2 years of age and were found to have an esotropia with an increased accommodative-convergence ratio. Since there was no significant hyperopia, echothiophate eyedrops 0.125% were prescribed. One drop was to be instilled into each eye at bedtime. Within several hours after the initial instillation of eyedrops the patients became highly excitable ("almost wild"), cried and screamed continuously, became extremely restless and jittery ("in almost constant body movement"), were unreasonable, and had some "convulsivelike movements"—probably tremors. The parents initially thought their child had "a bad dream" or a nightmare. The children remained uncontrollable for several hours. One child did not return to his normal personality until almost 12 hours later. Each child had improved by the next day, and thus the echothiophate eyedrops were again instilled at bedtime. The same acute toxic manifestations occurred within 2 hours and persisted for the greater part of the night. The association of eyedrops and reaction was then realized, and the therapy was discontinued. One patient subsequently had surgery for strabismus. A plasma sample for cholinesterase determination was obtained at the time of surgery. The level was normal.

An unusual response to drugs by patients with mongolism has been known. Benda[5] commented on the unusual reaction to insulin and to epinephrine (Adrenalin) when these drugs were used in tolerance tests for the study of carbohydrate metabolism in children with Down's syndrome. After insulin injection some mongoloids exhibited a prolonged period of sleepiness, sweating, fever, desire to urinate, and in some cases, tremor. After intravenous injection of epinephrine, two mongoloids showed immediate marked temporary reactions, such as extreme pallor, gagging, discomfort, fear, and accelerated pulse.

Atropine may cause an exaggerated pupil response or an abnormal systemic reaction after topical instillation.[6, 7]

Harris and Goodman[8] gave evidence that the increased sensitivity of patients with Down's syndrome to the cardioacceleratory effects of intravenous atropine constituted a pharmacogenetic abnormality that may result from the genetic imbalance imposed by an extra chromosome 21.

Until additional clinical and laboratory observations are made in more patients with Down's syndrome, the immediate toxic manifestations exhibited by these patients to echothiophate are tentatively considered hyperreactive in nature. It seemed worthwhile even at this preliminary stage to alert others to the possible reaction.

"Miotic-URI"

The second toxic manifestation that deserves attention and recognition I have labelled the "miotic-URI." I suspect it is more common than is realized.

Some children receiving either echothiophate or isoflurophate develop a persistent mild rhinorrhea. They have no other local or systemic signs of parasympathetic hyperactivity. These children are often subjected to many laboratory tests, drugs, and even antibiotics. They may be kept home from school for periods of time, or office appointments are cancelled because of the "chronic resistant cold."

The association between localized parasympathetic stimulation of the glands of the upper respiratory tract and the strong miotic usually has been overlooked by the pediatrician and by the ophthalmologist. Occasionally the pediatrician thought that the child suffered from an allergic rhinitis. Indeed, some of the children did have a history of allergies. The diagnosis of allergic rhinitis was eliminated, however, when symptoms disappeared on discontinuing the miotic therapy. In those children who have "miotic-URI" and are receiving isoflurophate, the possibility of an allergy to the medication was excluded, since the rhinorrhea reappeared when echothiophate eyedrops were substituted.

Certain toxic effects of anticholinesterase agents, such as rhinorrhea, sensation of chest constriction, cough, and dyspnea, may have no definite correlation with erythrocyte cholinesterase inhibition. In a study of 525 cases of industrial exposure to sarin, an anticholinesterase nerve gas, 83% of the patients had rhinorrhea, with only 0 to 10% reduction in the erythrocyte cholinesterase level.[9]

An awareness by the ophthalmologist and the pediatrician of the possible relationship between anticholinesterase eye medication and symptoms restricted to the upper respiratory tract will lead to prompt diagnosis and elucidation of this problem in children receiving strong miotic therapy.

REFERENCES

1. Roy, F. H., Hanna, C., and others: Irreversible miosis following long-term echothiophate (Phospholine) iodide use, J. Ped. Ophthal. **7**:46, 1970.
2. Jones, D. E. P., and Watson, D. M.: Angle-closure glucoma precipitated by the use of Phospholine iodide for esotropia in a child, Brit. J. Ophthal. **51**: 783, 1967.
3. Harrison, R.: Bilateral lens opacities associated with the use of di-isopropyl fluorophate eyedrops, Amer. J. Ophthal. **50**:153, 1960.
4. Axelsson, U., and Nyman, K-G: Side effects from use of long-acting cholinesterase inhibitors in young persons, Acta Ophthal. **48**:396, 1970.
5. Benda, C. E.: Down's syndrome: mongolism and its management, New York, 1969, Grune & Stratton, Inc.
6. McKusick, V. A.: Symposium on inborn errors of metabolism: mechanism in genetic diseases of man, Amer. J. Med. **22**:676, 1957.
7. Walsh, F. W.: Clinical Neuro-ophthalmology, ed. 2, Baltimore, 1957, The Williams and Wilkins Co.
8. Harris, W. S., and Goodman, R. M.: Hyper-reactivity of atropine in Down's syndrome, New Eng. J. Med. **279**:407, 1968.
9. Wills, J. H.: Toxicity of anticholinesterases and its treatment. In International encyclopedia of pharmacology and therapeutics, section 13, vol. 1: Anticholinesterase agents, New York, 1970, Pergamon Press, Inc., p. 387.

Chapter 3

Subconjunctival therapy

Philip P. Ellis, M.D.

Ophthalmologists have administered drugs by the subconjunctival route for decades. From an historic standpoint such types of drugs as antiseptics, local irritants, and osmotic agents have been injected subconjunctivally.[1] At the present time subconjunctival injections are used primarily to introduce drugs into the eye and also to achieve local anesthesia. A variety of medications, including antibiotics, corticosteroids, and mydriatics, may be administered by the subconjunctival method.

Varying opinions exist among ophthalmologists regarding the clinical usefulness of subconjunctival injections. Some employ the technique quite routinely, while others hold this method to offer no significant advantages over other methods of drug application.

ADVANTAGES

The apparent advantages of subconjunctival therapy are that high tissue levels and usually correspondingly high intraocular penetration of the drug may be obtained without many of the problems of systemic dosage required to achieve comparable drug levels. Because the corneal and conjunctival epithelial barrier is bypassed, drugs with poor lipoid solubility characteristics may be introduced into the eye by the subconjunctival route when satisfactory levels cannot be obtained by topical application. In certain instances subconjunctival drug administration may overcome the unreliability of some patients, nursing personnel problems, and so on. This is notably true with the use of subconjunctival repository corticosteroids where a therapeutic response may last for several weeks. Subconjunctival injections during or at the conclusion of surgery avoid the necessity of topical or systemic therapy in patients during the immediate postoperative period.

DISADVANTAGES

There is limited duration of effect of subconjunctival administration of aqueous, nonrepository preparations; therapeutic drug levels are usually achieved only for a few hours. Localized side reactions, including pain, redness, chemosis, and scar formation, may occur. Chemical iritis has occurred.[2] Brawny scleritis has been reported after subconjunctival administration of atropine.[3] Increased intraocular pressure may occur both from compression of the vascular channels and the intraocular effect of the medication, that is, corticosteroids. In the former case the effect is usually quite transient, whereas with the administration of respository corticosteroids the induced glaucoma may persist for several weeks. Sufficient amounts of the drug may be absorbed to produce systemic reactions, especially with subconjunctival administration of epinephrine and cocaine.

TECHNIQUES

Subconjunctival injections are easily given after topical anesthesia, with a short 25- or 27-gauge disposable needle attached to a tuberculin syringe. The conjunctiva is picked up with a forceps a few millimeters behind the limbus, and 0.3 ml. to 0.5 ml. of the medication is injected. It is advisable to select a site where the greatest effect is desired. For example, if one is using repository corticosteroids for the treatment of an inferior cyclitis, the medication should be placed in the lower subconjunctival space, since the greatest intraocular drug concentration is in the area adjacent to the site of injection.[4] Injections may be given at daily intervals; but because of local side reactions, they usually cannot be given more often than at 24-hour intervals. Some scar formation and partial obliteration of the potential subconjunctival space may occur with repeated subconjunctival administration so that it may not be possible to repeat the injections in the same site; after many injections increased difficulty is encountered in placing the medication. Most conjunctival medications produce some degree of irritation; procaine has been used as a diluent for certain irritating drugs to relieve this distress. Epinephrine has also been added to the subconjunctival solution to prolong drug effect by inhibiting conjunctival vascular absorption.[5]

Alternate techniques of injection have been advised, including the placement of the injection through the lids and the placement of the medication beneath Tenon's capsule. The latter technique was suggested by Swan, Crisman, and Bailey,[6] who observed more rapid and profound mydriasis when epinephrine was injected in sub-Tenon's (subcapsular) space than when injected subconjunctivally. These investigators maintain that subcapsular injections bring the drug into direct contact with the episcleral and limbic stroma, whereas with subconjunctival (subepithelial) injections the drug is in intimate approximation with conjunctival vessels and is rapidly carried off. The avascular Tenon's capsule separates the drug in the subcapsular space from conjunctival circulation. On the basis of this study, sub-Tenon's injections have been widely recommended.

INTRAOCULAR PENETRATION

Several opinions exist as to the exact manner in which subconjunctival medications penetrate the eye. The most generally held view is that the drug diffuses across the scleral stroma, which has permeability characteristics comparable to those of the corneal stroma. This would explain the very high concentrations of the water-soluble penicillins that may be obtained in the aqueous humor after subconjunctival injections. Alternatively, it has been suggested that the medication leaks out of the subconjunctival space into tears and enters the eye through the cornea.[7] While this hypothesis might explain the intraocular penetration of highly lipoid soluble nonpolar drugs, such as the corticosteroids, it does not explain the penetration of polar water-soluble agents, such as penicillins.

Harris[8] studied ocular tissue concentrations of labelled eserine salicylate following application to bare sclera. The results suggested that subconjunctival medications enter the corneal stroma through the limbus and subsequently cross the endothelium, which does not present nearly the same lipoid barrier as does the corneal epithelium. In our laboratory Hardy and Paterson[9] have arrived at a similar conclusion by studying the aqueous humor concentrations of labelled chloramphenicol after subconjunctival injection.

Antibiotics

Many studies have established that most antibiotics penetrate into the anterior chamber of the eye in good concentrations after subconjunctival administration.[5, 10-20] Notable among these studies is the work of Sorsby and Ungar,[21] who have demonstrated that antibiotics administered subconjunctivally at the time of or within a few hours after the inoculation of virulent strains of staphylococci were successful in preventing ocular destruction; but if the antibiotic was not given, a destructive endophthalmitis that responded poorly to any therapy developed within 24 hours. These studies suggest the two most useful applications of subconjunctival antibiotics: as a prophylaxis after surgery or injury and as an initial supplement to systemic antibiotic treatment of bacterial endophthalmitis.

Several studies indicate that subconjunctival injection of antibiotics at the end of surgery reduces the incidence of postoperative infection.[22-24] It should be pointed out that bacterial endophthalmitis may occur with the prophylactic subconjunctival antibiotic therapy even though the antibiotic coverage theoretically was effective against the offending organisms.[25] Also, the onset of a bacterial endophthalmitis may be obscured or delayed with this therapy.[26] McPherson, Presley, and Crawford[20] have suggested that antibiotics should be injected at the start of surgery to produce bacteriostasis of the anterior segment of the eye during the surgery.

As indicated above, most antibiotics enter the anterior chamber of the eye in high concentrations after subconjunctival administration. The apparent exceptions are the tetracyclines, ristocetin, streptomycin, and amphotericin B.[5, 14, 20, 27, 28] A recent study indicated that chloramphenicol did not penetrate into the anterior chamber after subconjunctival injection,[20] although earlier studies suggested that it did.[5, 13, 14]

Useful antibiotic levels usually do not persist in the aqueous humor for more than a few hours after subconjunctival administration.[2, 19] Repository penicillins do not penetrate into the aqueous humor in therapeutic concentrations after subconjunctival administration.[29] Because of the short duration of effect and also because of the infrequency with which subconjunctival antibiotics may be administered, their value in the treatment of bacterial endophthalmitis has been questioned.

Antibiotics are more effective against rapidly growing and dividing organisms that are present in the early phase of bacterial endophthalmitis. Following very high antibiotic concentrations, effective bacteriostasis may persist for many hours after the antibiotic has disappeared. For these reasons supplemental subconjunctival antibiotic therapy is indicated early in the treatment of bacterial endophthalmitis when there is severe involvement of the anterior segment of the eye.

Suggested dosages of subconjunctival antibiotics are: ampicillin, 50 mg.; bacitracin, 10,000 units; cephaloridine, 50 mg.; cephalothin, 50 mg.; chloramphenicol, 50 mg.; colistin, 20 mg.; gentamicin, 3 mg.; kanamycin, 10 to 20 mg.; methicillin, 50 to 100 mg.; penicillin G, 500,000 units; and polymyxin B, 5 to 10 mg.[30]

Corticosteroids

When corticosteroids first became available for ophthalmic use, they were given subconjunctivally as well as by other techniques.[31] It was soon appreciated that although injections of cortisone and hydrocortisone suspensions gave good therapeutic concentrations in the aqueous humor, almost equally high levels could be obtained with topical therapy. The suspending agent, hydroxypropyl methylcellulose, persisted in the subconjunctival space as a “puttylike” mass for several weeks or months.

This mass was therapeutically inactive. With the advent of repository corticosteroid preparations, the use of subconjunctival steroids has again become quite popular. The duration of therapeutic effects with repository corticosteroids appears to last from 1 to 6 weeks. Therapeutically active steroid has been demonstrated in the subconjunctival space 3 weeks after injection in a human being.[32] Repository corticosteroid therapy has been used in the treatment of severe anterior segment inflammatory disease. It has been advocated in the treatment of chronic cyclitis (pars planitis), and after glaucoma surgery, keratoplasty, and cataract surgery in eyes with smoldering iritis.[32-34] Steroid-induced glaucoma may occur with subconjunctival steroids as early as 10 days after the injection.[35] Because of the slow absorption of repository subconjunctival steroids, the glaucoma may persist for an extended time.

In the past 2 years subconjunctival injections of 4 mg. of aqueous dexamethasone in combination with topical corticosteroids and appropriate specific therapeutic agents have been advocated for the treatment of severe central stromal keratitis of the various causes.[36]

Mydriatics

The value of subconjunctival injection of mydriatic agents is well established.[37, 38] Various mixtures of epinephrine, phenylephrine, atropine, homatropine methylbromide, and cocaine have been advocated. The medications are sometimes effective in dilating resistant pupils and breaking posterior synechiae. It should be pointed out that injections of epinephrine, cocaine, and atropine may produce systemic side reactions.

Pralidoxime (Protopam) chloride, an antagonist of certain anticholinesterase agents, also has been injected subconjunctivally to produce mydriasis.[39] Treatment consists of topical instillation of echothiophate. After miosis, a subconjunctival injection of 0.1 to 0.2 ml. of 5% solution of aqueous pralidoxime chloride is given, followed by topical administration of 10% phenylephrine and 1% atropine.

Heparin

Recently the subconjunctival injection of heparin, 300 units daily, has been advocated for the treatment of certain peripheral corneal diseases thought to result from ischemic necrosis.[40] Included in this group of diseases are marginal, furrow, and gutter dystrophies, peripheral ring ulcers, Mooren's ulcer, chemical keratitis, and postoperative ischemic necrosis.

REFERENCES

1. Duke-Elder, S., editor: System of ophthalmology. The foundations of ophthalmology: heredity, pathology, diagnosis and therapeutics, vol. 7, St. Louis, 1962, The C. V. Mosby Co.

2. Records, R. E., and Ellis, P. P.: Subconjunctival antibiotic therapy in ophthalmology; with special considerations of the penicillins and cephalosporins, Trans. Pacif. Coast Otoophthal. Soc. **50**:179, 1969.
3. Swan, K. C., and Butler, J. B. V.: Brawny type of scleritis following subconjunctival injections, Trans. Pacif. Coast Otoophthal. Soc. **31**:111, 1950.
4. McCartney, H. J., Drysdale, I. O., and others: An autoradiographic study of the penetration of subconjunctivally injected hydrocortisone into the normal and inflamed rabbit eye, Invest. Ophthal. **4**:297, 1965.
5. Sorsby, A., Ungar, J., and Crick, R. P.: Aureomycin, chloramphenicol and terramycin in ophthalmology, Brit. Med. J. **2**:301, 1953.
6. Swan, K. C., Crisman, H. R., and Bailey, P. F., Jr.: Subepithelial versus subcapsular injections of drugs, Arch. Ophthal. **56**:26, 1956.
7. Wine, N. A., Gornal, A. G., and Basu, P. K.: The ocular uptake of subconjunctivally injected C^{14} hydrocortisone: I, time and major route of penetration in a normal eye, Amer. J. Ophthal. **58**:362, 1964.
8. Harris, J. E.: Problems in drug penetration. In Leopold, I. H., editor: Symposium on ocular therapy, vol. 3, St. Louis, 1968, The C. V. Mosby Co.
9. Hardy, R. G., and Paterson, C. A.: Ocular penetration of ^{14}C-labeled chloramphenicol following subconjunctival or sub-Tenon's injection, Amer. J. Ophthal. **71**:1307, 1971.
10. Struble, G. C., and Bellows, J. G.: Studies on the distribution of penicillin in the eye and its clinical application, J. A. M. A. **125**:685, 1944.
11. Leopold, I. H., and La Motte, W. O., Jr.: Penetration of penicillin in rabbit eyes with normal, inflamed and abraded corneas, Arch. Ophthal. 33:43, 1945.
12. Andrews, G. W. S.: Distribution of penicillin in the eye after subconjunctival injection, Lancet **1**:594, 1947.
13. Leopold, I. H., Nichols, A. C., and Vogel, D. W.: Penetration of chloramphenicol U. S. P. (Chloromycetin) into the eye, Arch. Ophthal. **44**:22, 1950.
14. Furgiuele, F. P., Sery, T. W., and Leopold, I. H.: Newer antibiotics: their intraocular penetration, Amer. J. Ophthal. **50**:614, 1960.
15. Kurose, Y., Sery, T. W., and Leopold, I. H.: Intraocular penetration of thiosporin, Amer. J. Ophthal. **57**:418, 1964.
16. Furgiuele, F. P.: New antibiotics: their intraocular penetration, part II, Amer. J. Ophthal. **58**:443, 1964.
17. Kurose, Y., and Leopold, I. H.: Intraocular penatration of ampicillin: I, animal experiments, Arch. Ophthal. **73**:361, 1965.
18. Furgiuele, F. P.: Ocular penetration and tolerance of gentamicin, Amer. J. Ophthal. **64**: 421, 1967.
19. Records, R. E., and Ellis, P. P.: The intraocular penetration of ampicillin, methicillin and oxacillin, Amer. J. Ophthal. **64**:135, 1967.
20. McPherson, S. D., Jr., Presley, G. D., and Crawford, J. R.: Aqueous humor assays of subconjunctival antibiotics, Amer. J. Ophthal. **66**:430, 1968.
21. Sorsby, A., and Ungar, J.: The control of experimental infections of the anterior chamber and of the vitreous by subconjunctival and retrobulbar injections of crystalline penicillin in doses of 1,000,000 units, Brit. J. Ophthal. **32**:873, 1948.
22. Pearlman, M. D.: Prophylactic subconjunctival penicillin and streptomycin after cataract extraction, Arch. Ophthal. **55**:516, 1956.
23. Kolker, A. E., Freeman, M. I., and Pettit, T. H.: Prophylactic antibiotics and postoperative endophthalmitis, Amer. J. Ophthal. **63**:434, 1967.
24. Cassady, J. R.: Prophylactic subconjunctival antibiotics following cataract extraction, Amer. J. Ophthal. **64**:1081, 1967.
25. Chalkley, T. H., and Shoch, D.: An evaluation of prophylactic subconjunctival antibiotic injection in cataract surgery, Amer. J. Ophthal. **64**:1084, 1967.
26. Aronstam, R.: Pitfalls of prophylaxis: alteration of postoperative infection by penicillin-streptomycin, Amer. J. Ophthal. **57**:312, 1964.

27. Abraham, R. K., and Burnett, H. H.: Tetracycline and chloramphenicol studies on rabbit and human eyes, Arch. Ophthal. **54**:641, 1955.
28. Green, W. R., Bennett, J. E., and Goos, R. D.: Ocular penetration of amphotericin B: a report of laboratory studies and a case report of post surgical cephalosporium endophthalmitis, Arch. Ophthal. **73**:769, 1965.
29. Records, R. E.: Subconjunctival injection of the repository penicillins: a comparative study of the intraocular penetration, Arch. Ophthal. **78**:380, 1967.
30. Ellis, P. P., and Smith, D. L.: Handbook of ocular therapeutics and pharmacology, ed. 3, St. Louis, 1969, The C. V. Mosby Co.
31. Leopold, I. H., Purnell, J. E., and others: Local and systemic cortisone and ocular disease, Amer. J. Ophthal. **34**:361, 1951.
32. Rodger, F. C.: Repository corticotherapy in ophthalmic theory and practice, Brit. J. Ophthal. **49**:298, 1965.
33. Coles, R. S., Krohn, D. L., and others: Depo-Medrol in treatment of inflammatory disease, Amer. J. Ophthal. **54**:407, 1962.
34. Kimura, S. J., and Hogan, M. J.: Chronic cyclitis, Arch. Ophthal. **71**:193, 1964.
35. Kalina, R. E.: Increased intraocular pressure following subconjunctival corticosteroid administration, Arch. Ophthal. **81**:788, 1969.
36. Aronson, S. B., and Moore, T. E., Jr.: Corticosteroid therapy in central stromal keratitis, Amer. J. Ophthal. **67**:873, 1969.
37. Flynn, F.: Mydriatic synergy: a note on the use of mydriatics by sub-conjunctival injection, Brit. J. Ophthal. **17**:298, 1933.
38. Newton, F. H.: Empirical treatment of uveitis, Arch. Ophthal. **14**:618, 1935.
39. Byron, H. M., and Posner, I.: Clinical evaluation of Protopam, Amer. J. Ophthal. **57**:409, 1964.
40. Aronson, S. B., Elliott, J. H., and others: Pathogenetic approach to therapy of peripheral corneal inflammatory disease, Amer. J. Ophthal. **70**:65, 1970.

Chapter 4

Virus therapy

Herbert E. Kaufman, M.D.

In the treatment of herpes simplex of the eye, it is usually relatively easy to manage dendritic epithelial defects with idoxuridine (IDU) or by other means. The treatment of stromal disease and iritis with corticosteroids and IDU, while often satisfactory, is prolonged, entails some hazard, and is far from ideal. Similarly, the problem of preventing recurrences of herpetic keratitis is one that has not been solved. New approaches to the understanding of these problems are developing, however, and although they may not be immediately applicable today, they are sufficiently important for us all to be aware of them.

One new approach to the prevention of recurrences of herpes infection has been through an understanding of the recently elaborated secretory antibody system. When we are infected with a virus, a variety of antibodies develop in our bloodstream. These are predominantly a large molecular antibody, gamma M antibody, and a smaller molecular gamma G antibody; these antibodies seem primarily responsible for our systemic immunity. Until recently, however, a number of problems related to virus resistance could not be explained by our understanding of these antibodies. When children were given dead polio virus vaccines systemically, they were resistant to polio in that they did not develop paralysis from virus travelling through the bloodstream to the brain. They did, however, remain susceptible to polio infection and could be infected by virus in the intestine, and they shed the virus even though they did not develop clinical disease. If these children received the oral Sabin vaccine, however, not only were they protected systemically, but the surface of the intestine was also protected, and these children could not be infected.

This study was supported in part by U. S. Public Health Service research grants EY-00007 and EY-00446 from the National Eye Institute, Bethesda, Maryland.

Similar considerations seem to apply in the case of vaccination against influenza. Systemic vaccination is not completely effective. Very small amounts of antigen given by nose drops or inhalation seem nearly as effective, or in some cases more effective, than systemic immunization, even though the level of circulating antibodies may be quite a bit lower.

Such observations are explained by the finding of a special secretory antibody on the surfaces of the body, including the mucous membrane of the eye, which seems to provide a unique type of protection to the eye and other surfaces. In response to local instillation of antigens, the plasma cells under the epithelial surfaces secrete a gamma A antibody. Although some of this appears in the bloodstream, much of it goes to the epithelial cells, where it appears to be conjugated with a special protein and secreted on to the mucosal surface, giving a local type of protection that is independent, in a general way, from systemic immunization.

In herpes simplex infections, Dr. Centifanto and associates[1] have found that there is in tears a gamma A antibody that is a neutralizing antibody for herpesvirus. This antibody can be stimulated in rabbits and men by the topical instillation of dead virus, and the stimulated eye responds more than the nonstimulated eye. The eyes also vary in their production of herpes antibodies from time to time. Such local antibodies might explain why individuals in whom herpes infection frequently recurs have high, stable circulating titers of neutralizing antibody but unknown quantities of locally protective antibody. Similarly, it might be possible to stimulate antibody production locally in the eye with eye drops containing dead virus antigen and to create a level of immunity and resistance that could prevent recurrences of this disease. Animal studies in rabbits in which herpes keratitis frequently recurs reveal, however, that these recurrences occur in the face of high tear antibody levels and that the stimulation of antibodies by the continued instillation of dead virus, while easily documented, does not prevent recurrences of the disease. It appears that although this antibody is capable of neutralizing the virus, other types of antibody are also produced that can coat the virus and partially protect it from the neutralizing effect of the gamma A antibody. Hope remains, however, that this system can be modified so that local vaccination by dead virus instilled in eye drops may sometimes produce a useful protection against virus disease—especially disease caused by herpesvirus or adenovirus.

Another approach to the control and prevention of virus disease is through interferon. A protein made by infected cells, interferon induces other cells to develop a broad protection against virus disease. Different viruses produce it at different levels and are susceptible to it in different

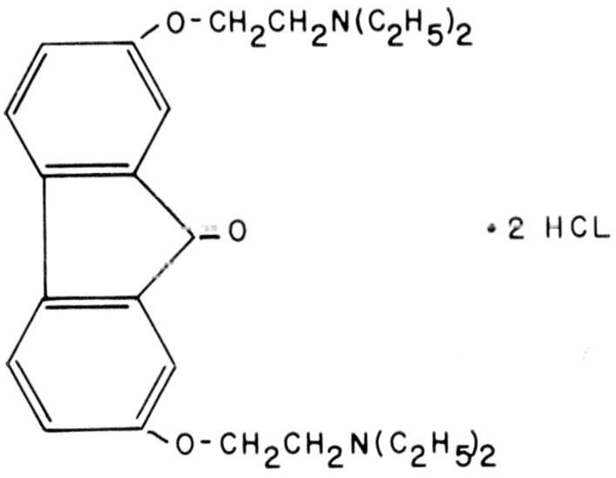

Fig. 4-1. Tilorone hydrochloride.

ways. Unfortunately, herpesvirus and adenovirus are poor stimulators of interferon and are quite resistant to interferon action. Nevertheless, compounds have been found that induce the host to produce interferon. One type is a long chain synthetic molecule that is chemically somewhat similar to the genetic material of an infecting virus and can fool the cell into producing interferon. This sythetic RNA has very low therapeutic activity, although this activity is significant in lower animals, and protects against infection for a limited period of time. Present evidence, however, suggests that this double-stranded RNA is much more effective in lower animals than in primates and man, and this seems to be true of similar long chain carboxylic acids, pyran, and chemically related substances.

A totally new type of interferon inducer called tilorone hydrochloride (Fig. 4-1) has recently been developed. This is a small molecular weight compound that is quite different from the other interferon inducers, and there was good reason to believe that this might be effective in man because of its different chemical nature. We administered 1,000 mg. per day of this drug to volunteers and measured interferon in a human skin and muscle tissue culture system, with vesicular stomatitis virus as the indicator virus. No interferon was found in the blood. Giving this drug topically, however, produced troubles that we did not anticipate. Although the drug was exceedingly well tolerated, one drop of 200 mg./ml. of drug given in saline produced no signs or symptoms for 7 to 10 days. Thereafter, with only one drop a day, the subjects began to complain of haloes around lights and blurred vision. Corneal edema was seen on biomicroscopy in the epithelium. The stroma and other areas of the eye were completely normal. It soon became apparent that the drug was accumulating in the epithelium, and administration of the drug was stopped. Haloes and blurred vision persisted; two of our subjects who were used to psychedelic phenomena from other causes en-

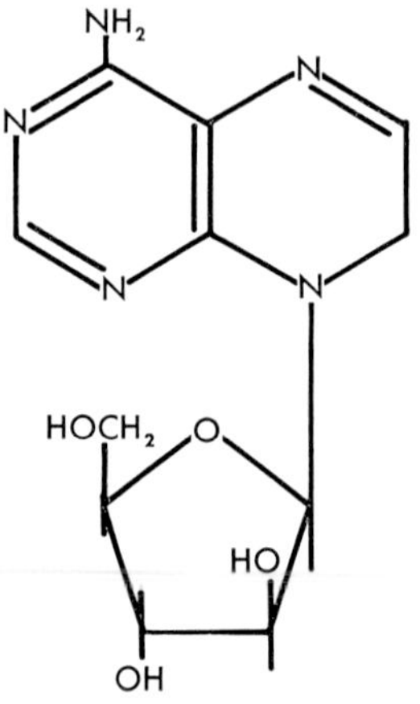

Fig. 4-2. Adenine arabinoside.

joyed the visual sensations. The subjects had halo vision and drug deposits for approximately 2 months after a short course of drug administration, although throughout this time no interferon was found in the tears. Hope still remains that it may be possible to mobilize the interferon system in man in some useful way, but this has not yet been established.

Another fascinating approach to the control of virus disease with broad-spectrum agents involved the drug isoprinosine (inosine; dimethylaminoisopropanol 1:3 complex, *P*-acetamidobenzoate). This is a very simple and nontoxic compound chemically related to one of the ordinary nucleoside bases used by the body in building genetic material. In animals it is said to promote learning, to reduce some of the changes of aging, and to have a definite effect against virus disease. Our own studies in rabbits confirm that it has an effect against herpetic iritis, offering some promise that such an effect might be seen in man. This drug, which seems relatively innocuous, appears to act by inhibiting the takeover of the cell by the virus genetic material—inhibiting the readout of the virus nucleic acid. Our present studies in man are preliminary but suggest that such a drug may have a significant clinical effect. These studies are now in progress, and we hope shortly to have a significant clinical series.

The final new approach to the treatment of deep virus infections involves the use of newer antimetabolites. Adenine arabinoside is a unique type of antimetabolite (Fig. 4-2). Unlike most of those with which we are familiar, it has little tendency to produce bone marrow deficiency and hematologic abnormalities. In rabbits we have shown that it is active against herpetic iritis induced by virus placed directly into the anterior chamber. It is active when given either systemically or subconjunctivally, and this activity is seen with no apparent systemic toxicity. IDU and trifluorothymidine, which are active topically, present relatively little systemic hazard in part because they are rapidly metabolized. This very property, however, and the rapid breakdown in vascularized tissues make these compounds relatively unsatisfactory for the treatment of deeper infection. Adenine arabinoside is not only more slowly metabolized, but its major metabolic product, hypoxantine arabinoside, is also an effective antiviral agent. We have used this compound subconjunctivally in a couple of patients; and although there may be some effect on the disease, the effect is uncertain. Further trial certainly seems justified, however; and even if compounds such as adenine arabinoside and isoprinosine in themselves are not sufficiently active, it is possible that using combinations of relatively nontoxic substances may permit effective therapy.

This discussion has outlined a variety of new approaches to the control of virus disease, ranging from the mobilization of natural defenses, such as the secretory antibody system and interferon, to the use of totally new kinds of drugs with activity in animal systems against the kinds of viruses we worry most about. These approaches offer great possibilities for the future, and I hope that we will all be using at least one of them soon.

REFERENCE

1. Centifanto, Y. M., Little, J. M., and Kaufman, H. E.: Relationship between virus chemotherapy, secretory antibody formation and recurrent herpetic disease, Ann. N. Y. Acad. Sci. 173:649, 1970.

Chapter 5

Points in the treatment of bacterial corneal ulcers

Frederick H. Theodore, M.D.

Surprisingly little is available, either in books or elsewhere in the literature, in regard to the actual management of bacterial ulcers of the cornea. As Dr. Henry F. Allen[1] has mentioned in his notes for graduate students, while there is considerable information available concerning laboratory studies of various antibiotics, these studies are often based on animal experiments. Even where human studies are involved, the ophthalmologist does not get a clear picture of just how to proceed in the occasional case that he encounters. For this reason it was thought worthwhile to offer a specific approach to the treatment of bacterial infections of the cornea based on considerable practical experience in this field that goes back many years.[1a] During this time a number of practical points and other observations of some importance have been noted. Certain aspects of this approach, such as the office use of subconjunctival antibiotics and the topical use of specially prepared high concentrations of indicated antibiotics, have up to now apparently not been emphasized.

No one needs to be told about the urgency of bacterial corneal ulcers, which despite mild beginnings may within the course of 24 to 48 hours spread extensively, develop hypopyon, and thus become serious ophthalmic problems. As such, any corneal infection, especially bacterial, once diagnosed or even suspected must be considered an ophthalmic emergency requiring urgent attention.

Success in such treatment depends on early bacterial diagnosis, immediate intensive treatment, and daily observation.

DIAGNOSIS

It is not the province of this chapter to detail the various clinical clues in the diagnosis of corneal infections.[2] One must, however, emphasize the great value of early, exact microbiologic diagnosis in the treatment of each individual case.[3] In order to facilitate early diagnosis, scrape smears and cultures of the corneal ulcer should be performed in the ophthalmologist's office before definitive treatment is begun. This is a medical procedure to be performed by the ophthalmologist. Although topical anesthetics that contain preservatives may theoretically inhibit the growth of germs, their use is advisable. Cultures should be made with a platinum or other type of spatula and a sterile cotton applicator. The base of the ulcer should be gently scraped. The applicator should first be moistened with broth before touching the ulcer. Both are inoculated into blood agar, Sabouraud's agar, and a suitable broth media. Allen's experience has been that liquid media often gives positive cultures where solid media show no growth. My own experience has been that either type may be negative when the other type is positive. It is entirely feasible for every ophthalmologist to store some glucose broth (with or without refrigeration) in his office for such emergencies.

Smears of the ulcer should be examined immediately by the ophthalmologist in order to obtain early clues as to the direction of treatment and choice of antibiotics. Even if Gram stain is not available, the use of gentian violet or any other similar dye will offer morphologic information concerning the possible bacterium or other microorganism present. Examination of such a smear, *if positive,* has the following additional advantages: (1) it saves the 24 to 48 hours of time that bacterial growth requires; (2) it saves the 2 to 12 days that fungal cultures may require before becoming positive; (3) it may be the only positive finding if cultures do not grow because of the prior antibiotic treatment or other reasons; and finally, (4) it is proof that any microorganism grown on culture is not a contaminant.

It should be emphasized that careful scrapings for microbiologic purposes are never harmful. Actually, such mechanical removal of necrotic material appears to enhance the effectiveness of antibiotics used in treatment.

Two further points in regard to cultures are important. First, a culture of the conjunctiva, while also desirable, must never be considered as a substitute for a corneal culture when a corneal ulcer is present. It is not the same thing, and its results may be entirely misleading. Second, the ophthalmologist must keep in constant touch with the laboratory concerning reports and antibiotic sensitivity tests. If left to the normal course of events, many days may elapse before urgently needed

Table 5-1. Subconjunctival injections of antibiotics

Penicillin G	250,000 to 1,000,000 units
Methicillin	150 to 200 mg.
Ampicillin	50 to 250 mg.
Lincomycin (Lincocin)	150 mg.
Erythromycin (Ilotycin)	100 mg.
Cephaloridine (Loridine)	100 mg.
Bacitracin	10,000 units
Neomycin	250 to 500 mg.
Streptomycin	50 to 100 mg.
Chloramphenicol sodium succinate	50 to 100 mg.
Polymyxin B	10 mg.
Colistin (Coly-Mycin)	15 to 37.5 mg.
Gentamicin (Garamycin)	10 to 20 mg.
Cephalothin (Keflin)	50 to 100 mg.
Carbenicillin	100 mg.

information is finally on the record. Unless the laboratory is alerted, such delays are the rule rather than the exception.

TREATMENT

The author's basic approach to the treatment of bacterial ulcers consists of subconjunctival injections of antibiotics in the office prior to hospitalization and the intensive use of concentrated solutions of indicated antibiotics in the hospital. Systemic antibiotics appear to be less important in such treatment.

Standard antibiotics, such as penicillin, neomycin (Mycifradin) sulfate, lincomycin (Lincocin), and gentamicin, are stocked in the office or should be readily obtainable from a nearby source.

Subconjunctival antibiotics

A positive smear revealing cocci of any type indicates the initial use of penicillin or lincomycin, in addition to neomycin. A slide showing bacilli, especially if gram-negative, indicates that the initial thrust of treatment should be against organisms like *Pseudomonas,* for which gentamicin, neomycin, and a covering dose of lincomycin are indicated. If the slide is negative or inconclusive, the entire antibacterial spectrum should be covered by using penicillin, lincomycin, and gentamicin. Dosages are given as indicated in Table 5-1. The patient should be warned that hemorrhages and pain may follow such injections in severely inflamed eyes. Experience has led me to place great value on subconjunctival therapy.[4]

The technique is a simple one. After preliminary topical anesthetics, those antibiotics readily diluted with 2% lidocaine (Xylocaine), such as neomycin, lincomycin, and gentamicin, are then injected subconjunctivally or under Tenon's capsule. Pencillin may be available in quantities small enough to be readily diluted with lidocaine. Otherwise, it is better to dilute it with sterile water or saline solution and inject lidocaine subconjunctivally in a new area before the injection of penicillin, or else to inject the penicillin into an area where the other antibiotics already have been injected. Although it is preferable to inject meperidine (Demerol) intramuscularly in the hospital to help relieve pain and anxiety, this procedure is not advisable in the office. Meperidine may incapacitate the patient to such an extent that getting him to the hospital later becomes a problem.

The advantages of immediate subconjunctival injections in the office should be apparent. The injection is done by the ophthalmologist himself and avoids the many hours lost while the patient is being admitted and getting a general work-up before definitive treatment is finally begun.

Subsequent injections during the course of treatment may be performed an additional 2 or 3 times, depending on the progress of the patient and the status of the conjunctiva, which in severe infections may become very hemorrhagic. The choice of antibiotics for such follow-up injections is governed by later laboratory findings and the clinical course of the disease. If the patient is doing well, the use of antibiotics used successfully so far should not be abandoned completely just because in-vitro laboratory tests indicate other choices.

The ophthalmologist must always inquire concerning possible allergies, especially to penicillin. If any question exists, a drop of diluted penicillin may first be instilled in the eye. If there is a specific history, the drug should not be used. Likewise, related drugs should be avoided if other antibiotics can be substituted.

Concentrated solutions of antibiotics for topical use

The choice of antibiotics commercially available to the ophthalmologist is not only limited, but diminishing. At present, only neomycin-polymyxin mixtures, gentamicin, and chloramphenicol can be purchased already prepared for use. Some of the tetracyclines (Aureomycin, Achromycin and Terramycin) are no longer available as commerically prepared eye drops. Furthermore, commercial solutions of neomycin and chloramphenicol (Chloromycetin) are relatively weak (in low concentration). Thus, for optimal results most corneal ulcers require therapy with antibiotics that are either not commercially obtainable or, if obtainable, not concentrated enough for most effective use.

It is my firm conviction that the frequent and intensive use of freshly prepared concentrated solutions of those specific antibiotics indicated in the individual case are always well tolerated over the 2- to 3-week period of intensive treatment needed. Preparation should be per-

Table 5-2. Topical drop therapy

	Concentrations used
Penicillin G	100,000 to 250,000 units/cc.
Methicillin	50 to 100 mg./cc.
Lincomycin (Lincocin)	50 to 150 mg./cc.
Bacitracin	10,000 units/cc.
Polymyxin B	5 to 10 mg./cc.
Colistin (Coly-Mycin)	7.5 mg./cc.
Gentamicin (Garamycin)	3 to 10 mg./cc.
Cephalothin (Keflin)	50 to 100 mg./cc.
Ampicillin	100 mg./cc.
Cephaloridine (Loridine)	50 to 100 mg./cc.
Chloramphenicol	5 mg./cc.
Neomycin (Mycifradin)	50 to 100 mg./cc.
Streptomycin	50 to 100 mg./cc.
Erythromycin (Ilotycin)	50 mg./cc.
Carbenicillin (Geopen)	100 mg./cc.

formed by the ophthalmologist, or by a nurse using his directions, in order to ensure sterility.[5, 6] Very few hospital pharmacies can be relied upon in regard to sterility where "homemade solutions" are compounded. Table 5-2 lists the concentrations of such antibiotics so used.

Untoward results are limited to allergy and irritation. Allergy, however, is related essentially to the drug used, not to its concentration, and is recognizable by the characteristic signs of allergic dermatoconjunctivitis with eczema of the eyelids. Surprisingly little irritation occurs with these strong solutions. When drug irritation does occur, it usually follows the use of neomycin and streptomycin, and is manifested by a fine punctate keratitis that disappears when the drug is either discontinued or its concentration lessened. In fact, no serious untoward result has occurred in the course of over 20 years of experience with such concentrated solutions.

Where original smears have given clues to the diagnosis, the same antibiotics used for subconjunctival injections are prescribed. If smears are negative, a principle similar to that used in choosing the subconjunctival antibiotics used initially is observed. Penicillin, lincomycin, and gentamicin are prescribed. Lincomycin is particularly recommended because of the excellent tolerance of the eye to its use and because it is stable and does not require refrigeration. Neomycin similarly is stable and does not require refrigeration, but may be more irritating, as noted above. This irritation also has been noted in other eye conditions after the prolonged use of weak neomycin solutions such as neomycin, or even in neomycin-steroid mixtures. The choice of topical antibiotics used later in the course of therapy is, of course, governed by the results of laboratory studies, the tolerance of the patient to the regime, and the clinical course of the disease.

The drugs are usually administered every hour day and night, all at the same time. As improvement occurs, the drugs are given every 2 hours at night, and still less later on. Theoretically, it might be better to give the different drops every 15 to 30 minutes, but this requires special nurses.

Daily observation

Careful daily observation of a patient with a corneal ulcer is as important as exact diagnosis and intensive treatment. Such examinations should include daily slit-lamp studies, both before and after staining with fluorescein, and careful notes, including drawings, of the daily status. It is only by this careful approach that the earliest indications of conditions requiring changes in treatment are recognized. Unless the records include diagrams, it is surprising how the busy ophthalmologist forgets the exact extent of the lesion he has seen only a day before. Even if the lesion is the same in size, notation as to the intensity of the fluorescein staining gives valuable clues as to progress in the eyes that otherwise appear extremely inflamed and little improved.

Early in the treatment of severe corneal ulcers it is difficult to judge progress and to ascertain how the patient is responding to the treatment. However, one must remember that an ulcer that has been getting steadily worse before treatment must first stop getting worse before it begins to improve. Therefore, at this stage, *if the ulcer is not getting worse, it is actually getting better.*

It is easy enough to institute intensive treatment for a corneal ulcer; it is far more difficult to decide when such intensive therapy is no longer necessary. It is my firm conviction, based on a number of cases where such treatment was stopped too soon, that it is *better to overtreat than to undertreat a corneal ulcer.* Even if check-up corneal cultures, which should be repeated every 3 to 4 days, show no growth, it is important to remember that deep in the corneal stroma there may be nests of viable bacteria. For this reason intensive treatment must be kept up for at least 10 days or 2 weeks in almost every case. However, as improvement continues, as indicated by such findings as clearing of the hypopyon, the general appearance of the ulcer with and without staining, the disappearance of conjunctival discharge, and subjective signs, topical drug treatment is lessened by making instillations less frequently (every 2 hours during the day and less often at night) and by using lower concentrations of antibiotics. Even after the patient has been discharged from the hospital, moderately intensive treatment is still in order.

In general, the use of corticosteroids should be avoided throughout the entire period of therapy. This is particularly true when dealing with

Pseudomonas or *Proteus* infections. In an apparently "cured" corneal ulcer caused by *Pseudomonas*, after 3 check-up cultures that were completely negative, the patient was given three injections of intravenous typhoid vaccine for severe iritis. These proved ineffectual. On this basis, the patient was given 3 drops of 0.1% dexamethasone daily while he was still on antibiotic regime of neomycin, polymyxin, and colistin, every 2 hours. Within a week he returned with a *Pseudomonas* ulcer worse than the one he had had originally. Other similar cases have been reported by Burns[7] and others. The individual resistance of each patient and each germ is different. It is thus wrong to assume that there is any fixed antibiotic dosage regime (antibiotic-steroid mixture) that will overcome the individual bacterium's "rejuvenation" by corticosteroids. In some patients, after check-up cultures have become negative, the cautious use of steroids covered by ample antibiotics (not fixed antibiotic-steroid combinations) may become necessary.

It is important to ensure good mydriasis with atropine in the early treatment of corneal ulcers. Posterior synechiae and pupillary occlusion following lack of dilation may result in such severe secondary glaucoma as to vitiate all the benefits of successful antiinfective therapy.

Finally, a point of some importance arises when the treating ophthalmologist cannot see the patient for a few days and requires a substitute. In order to be able to gauge progress correctly when he actually assumes responsibility, the second ophthalmologist should see the patient with the first physician the day before he takes over. Otherwise, he may not be in a position to appreciate and treat the changes that may subsequently occur.

REFERENCES

1. Allen, H. F.: Management of bacterial corneal ulcers, Harvard Medical School and Massachusetts Eye and Ear Infirmary. Privately published.
1a. Allen, H. F.: Current status of prevention, diagnosis, and management of bacterial corneal ulcers, Ann. Ophthal. **3**:235, 1971.
2. Theodore, F. H.: Clinical diagnosis of central corneal ulcers, Eye Ear Nose Throat Monthly **42**:82, 1963.
3. Theodore, F. H.: Slide diagnosis of central corneal ulcers, Eye Ear Nose Throat Monthly **42**:66, 1963.
4. Theodore, F. H.: Complications After Cataract Surgery, Boston, 1965, Little, Brown and Co., p. 76.
5. Theodore, F. H.: Contamination of eye solutions, Amer. J. Ophthal. **34**:1764, 1951.
6. Theodore, F. H., and Feinstein, R. R.: Practical suggestions for the preparation and maintenance of sterile ophthalmic solutions, Amer. J. Ophthal. **5**:656, 1952.
7. Burns, R. P.: Pseudomonas aeruginosa keratitis: mixed infections of the eye, Amer. J. Ophthal. **67**:257, 1969.

Chapter 6

Plasma expanders and lytic agents in ophthalmology

David Shoch, M.D., Ph.D.

The problem of arterial and venous occlusion of the retina remains perplexing and frustrating to the ophthalmologist. Fortunately, most of the branch arterial occlusions are embolic in nature, and these emboli often migrate spontaneously to more peripheral and thus less destructive positions. Also, one may occasionally be able to effect the dislocation of an occlusion by reduction of the intraocular pressure by means of paracentesis, massage, or hyperosmotic agents.

Unfortunately, most central artery occlusions and all venous occlusions are thrombotic in nature. There is no hope of rapid spontaneous resolution, and the measures noted above are not of any help.

In some cases anticoagulants may be useful, and since these can be easily controlled, they are used quite commonly in the treatment of thrombosis of retinal vessels.[1, 2] However, one would like to have available an agent that would prevent the propagation of a clot and dissolve one that was already present. Several such substances have recently become available and, as with most new drugs, have both promise and shortcomings.

Before discussing these it may be useful to review quickly current thought on the initiating mechanisms of thrombus formation[3] and dissolution, which are outlined as follows:

A. Formation
   1. Injury to endothelial wall with production of positive injury potential (release of ADP?)
   2. Attraction of negatively charged platelets to site of injury
   3. Aggregation of platelets (white thrombus)

4. Entrapment of fibrinogen and erythrocytes in thrombus (red thrombus)
5. Conversion of fibrinogen to fibrin (clot)

B. Dissolution—by conversion of entrapped profibrinolysin (plasminogen) to fibrinolysin (plasmin)

Although there are many factors involved, such as blood sludging, hereditary anomalies of coagulation, blood volume, dehydration, and so on, the major cause of thrombus formation is injury to the endothelial wall of the vessel. This permits or causes the adherence of platelets at the point of insult. Indeed, this is probably the normal mechanism for plugging small defects in vessels. It is only when the number of platelets adhering to the injury becomes very large that a thrombus is formed.

There are two explanations at this time for the adherence of platelets to damaged endothelium. Jorgensen and Borchgrevink[4] are the chief proponents of the theory that local release of adenosine diphosphate (ADP) by the injured endothelium causes platelet agglutination. This has been documented by many other observers. However, Sawyer[5] and his coworkers feel that platelet agglutination comes about through a change from the normal negative potential of the endothelial wall to a local, positive injury potential that attracts the negatively charged platelets. In any case, a platelet aggregate forms—the so-called white thrombus. Note that up to this stage blood coagulation is not involved, and indeed platelet aggregation can occur even in the presence of high blood levels of heparin or bishydroxycoumarin. The actual mechanism of blood coagulation is rather complicated, but suffice it to say that in the presence of thrombin the fibrinogen that is trapped in the interstices of the platelet mass is converted to fibrin and entraps erythrocytes, forming the so-called red thrombus. The slower the rate of blood flow past the thrombus, the greater will be the number of red blood cells in the clots. This is why venous occlusions are usually composed of red thrombi.

Therapeutic measures for clots take several routes: interference with platelet deposition and aggregation, interference with erythrocyte clumping, interference with the fibrinogen to fibrin process, or finally actual dissolution of the fibrin already present. Some possible therapies for thrombosis are:

A. Inhibition of platelet deposition and aggregation—dextran
B. Inhibition of erythrocyte aggregation—dextran
C. Decrease of blood viscosity by siliconization of vessel wall—dextran
D. Interference with fibrinogen to fibrin conversion
   1. Inhibition of prothrombin formation in liver—bishydroxycoumarin
   2. Inhibition of thrombin-fibrinogen reaction—heparin

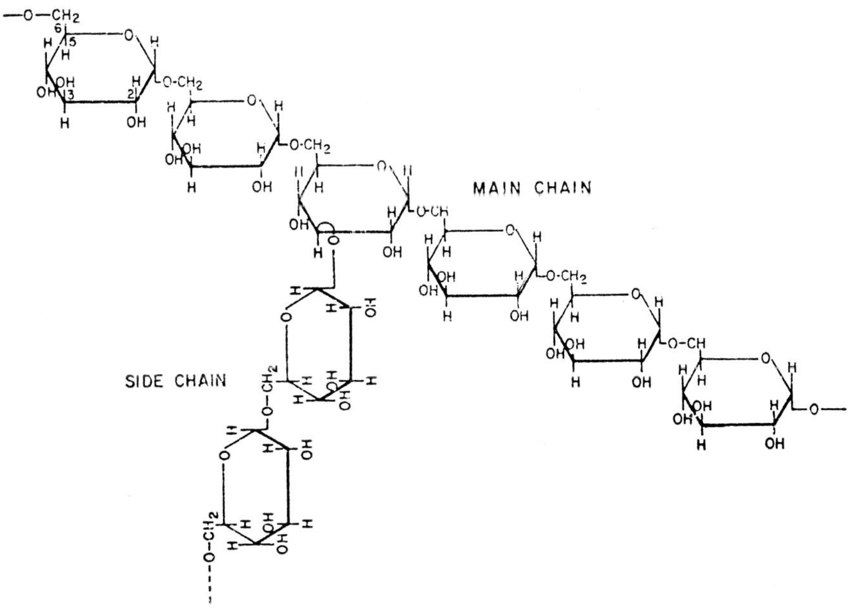

Fig. 6-1. Structural formula of dextran. (From Evarts, C. M.: Low molecular weight dextran, Med. Clin. N. Amer. **51**:1285, 1967.)

E. Activation of intrinsic profibrinolysin to fibrinolysin
   1. Streptokinase
   2. Urokinase

Interference with fibrinogen-fibrin transformation may be effected by heparin, which in the presence of a cofactor retards or prevents thrombin-fibrinogen interaction, or by bishydroxycoumarin and its analogs, which interfere with the production of prothrombin in the liver. As noted above, both these agents are commonly used in ophthalmology and will not be discussed further here. However, several new agents are available that act on the platelet aggregate or on the fibrin clot itself. These are discussed in this chapter.

PLASMA EXPANDERS

The term "plasma expanders" can be applied to any agent that increases the blood volume. Obviously this can include such transient volume expanders as saline, dextrose, and so on. However, generally it is restricted to solutions of large molecular weight; substances that have an oncotic pressure similar to that of plasma. For practical purposes there are three such substances: plasma (or whole blood), albumin, and dextran. It is the latter that concerns us here. Dextran is a glucose polymer synthesized from sucrose by many bacteria but most commonly by *Leuconostoc mesenteroides* (Fig. 6-1). As formed, it has a molecular weight of about one million. It is then hydrolyzed and fractionated to produce the lower molecular weight commercial dextran.[6] This was first used as a plasma volume expander in 1945 by Gronwall and Ingelman.[7] However, in 1959 Borgstrom and others[8] demonstrated that the thrombus formation in the ligated femoral vein of rabbits could be counteracted by the administration of low molecular weight (10,000) dextran. This was rapidly confirmed by other workers, both experimentally and clinically. That dextran does have an antithrombotic effect is established beyond doubt, but the mechanism of this effect is still uncertain. It was originally thought that it operated simply through expansion of the plasma volume and hemodilution. This does not seem tenable since other plasma expanders such as albumin do not have such an effect. Therefore other mechanisms were searched for. In 1957 a paper appeared[9] that showed that dextran adheres to formed elements of the blood; and in 1964 Bloom and associates[10] proposed that this adherence, plus the coating of the vascular endothelium, prevented intravascular thrombosis. Apparently the dextran deposited on the intima decreases the positive injury potential and thus diminishes the attraction of negatively charged platelets, which, as noted above, is the initial step in thrombus formation. The possible mechanisms of the action of dextran can be summarized as follows:

1. Plasma volume expansion
2. Alteration of positive injury potential
3. Alteration of platelet adhesiveness
4. Alteration of erythrocyte adhesiveness
5. Coating of endothelial wall

Unfortunately, retinal thromboses are rarely seen at their onset, and therefore the stage of platelet aggregation is long past in a clinical occlusion. However, there is some evidence that dextran also causes repulsion of erythrocytes, and this may inhibit the prolongation of a red thrombus. Further, the coating effect of dextran is long lasting, and this may cause a decrease in blood viscosity. It is well documented that increased blood viscosity tends to favor thrombus formation and expansion.

In any case, even though the mechanism of action of dextran is as yet in doubt, there is evidence that it is useful in thrombotic disease. For example, Gilroy and associates,[11] in a well-documented study, have shown that in patients with acute cerebral infarction mortality and morbidity can be reduced by administering dextran 40 intravenously for 3 days. Unfortunately, the evidence for the use of this material in ophthalmology is less convincing. The few papers that have appeared [12, 13] have no control studies, and in most cases other medications were used concomitantly, which confuses the data.

Finally, some caution must be exercised with the use of dextran, since renal failure has been reported after the use of low molecular weight dextran.[14] In addition, there is also some evidence that dextran can potentiate the effect of simultaneously given heparin. For this reason we feel that at this time dextran therapy should be limited to those patients whose only eye is involved in a vascular occlusion and who are not being treated with heparin.

As has been pointed out, dextran would be most effective as a prophylactic drug to prevent thrombi formation, since it acts on the initial stage of thrombus formation, that is, platelet and red blood cell aggregation. However, we cannot as yet identify those persons who are thrombus-prone, and we are therefore limited to treating thrombi that are already formed and are causing obvious clinical signs. For these it would be ideal to have a drug that could dissolve the thrombus that is already formed. There are such drugs, one available commercially and the other still experimental. These are the so-called fibrinolytic agents—fibrinolysin and urokinase, respectively.

Again before proceeding it might be wise to discuss normal fibrinolytic activity in the blood. Obviously this must exist to dissolve the microthrombi that form at sites of minimal injury to endothelium. This activity begins with the presence of a plasma globulin termed "plasminogen" that is present in a concentration of 0.1 to 0.2 mg./ml. The tissues contain an activator that converts this plasminogen to plasmin, a proteolytic enzyme that dissolves fibrin. Plasminogen is always present in the interstices of a thrombus and is then activated to form plasmin, which then dissolves the fibrin that enmeshes it.

The activator apparently arises from endothelial cells of the microcirculation so that capillary thrombi are rapidly cleared, but large-vessel thrombi persist much longer because of the paucity of activator present. The first pharmacologic approach, therefore, was to introduce into the circulation a plasminogen activator to raise the endogenous fibrinolytic activity. One of the most active of such activators is streptokinase, an enzyme elaborated by hemolytic streptococci.[15]

FIBRINOLYSIN

Fibrinolysin, or plasmin, (available commercially as Thrombolysin or Actase) is prepared from profibrinolysin (plasminogen), which is extracted and separated from other protein fractions in human plasma. It is then activated by the addition of streptokinase, an enzyme elaborated by hemolytic streptococci. There is some evidence that the activity of fibrinolysin is actually dependent on streptokinase activation of endogenous profibrinolysin.[16, 17] That fibrinolysin is effective in vitro is unquestioned; its activity in vivo is less solidly documented. Clots do tend to lyse spontaneously, and one must be conservative in evaluating the effectiveness of this material. However, there are occasional reports of the successful use of fibrinolysin in retinal occlusion.[18]

One such report[19] is documented by angiofluorography that shows normalization of the angiograms 2 hours after infusion of a streptokinase solution. Nevertheless, the evidence for benefit from fibrinolysis in retinal occlusion is sparse. Zweng and associates[19a] in their recent book state: "Fibrinolysin therapy was no better than placebo therapy in the treatment of retinal vein occlusion insofar as improvement in vision was concerned." Fibrinolysin has other drawbacks in that it occasionally produces pyrogenic reactions, and many patients have circulating antistreptokinase from previous streptococcal infections that would reduce the effectiveness of any particular dose. Finally, streptokinase is a bacterial product; so there is a measurable risk of antigenicity. For these reasons, attention turned several years ago to urokinase, a naturally occurring plasminogen activator present in human urine.[20]

UROKINASE

Although urokinase is not as yet commercially available, it seems to hold promise. It is a protein with a molecular weight of about 53,000 and has now been crystallized and standardized so that one mg. is equivalent to 35,000 CTA units.* Although it is a protein, it appears to be nonantigenic. Its usefulness in pulmonary embolism is well established.[21, 22] Its effectiveness in retinal occlusion is now being investigated. Zweng and associates[1] found little benefit from its use in eight patients with central artery occlusion but did find fluorescein-documented improvement in three of five patients with branch artery occlusion. Of eight patients with central vein occlusions, three improved, two got worse, and three remained the same. We have now begun to treat a series of patients in our clinic with the cooperation of Dr. H. C. Kwaan of the Department of Medicine.

Urokinase must be given intravenously, the initial loading dose being 2,000 CTA units. This same dose is given every hour for 4 to 6 hours, and the fibrinolytic activity is monitored by the euglobulin-lysis time.

Six patients have been treated thus far with urokinase; five had arterial occlusions and one had a venous occlusion. Two representative results are illustrated below.

Fig. 6-2, *A* shows a central retinal artery occlusion in the left eye of a young female who fortunately had a cilioretinal artery that preserved her macula. As is evident from the photograph, the whole retina except the perimacular area is edematous. Fig. 6-2, *B* is the angiogram done at

*CTA, Committee on Thrombolytic Agents of the National Heart Institute.

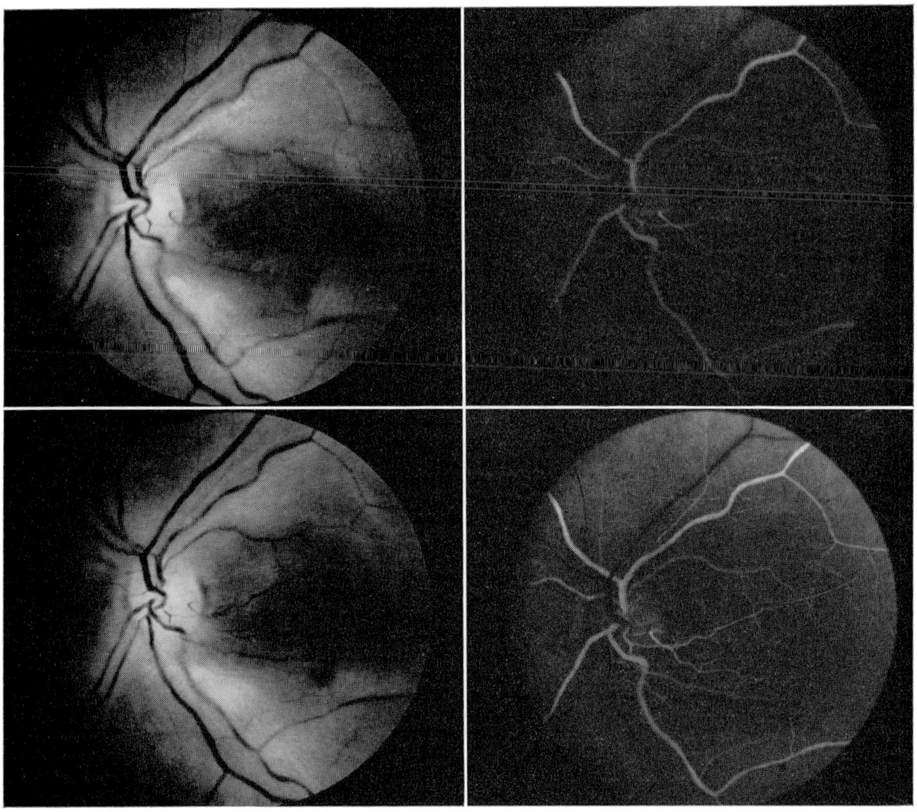

Fig. 6-2. A, Appearance of fundus of patient with a central retinal artery occlusion with an intact cilioretinal artery. **B,** Angiogram taken at initial visit. **C,** Appearance of fundus 24 hours after administration of urokinase. **D,** Fluoroangiogram 24 hours after administration of urokinase.

this time, showing the rather poor filling of the vessels. This is in the arterial phase. Fig. 6-2, *C* is the fundus photographed 24 hours after administration of urokinase. The edema seems to be a little less, but there is not a great deal of difference between this and Fig. 6-2, *A*. However, Fig. 6-2, *D*, taken at approximately the same time after administration of fluorescein, shows that there is much better filling of the arterial tree.

Fig. 6-3, *A* shows an occlusion of the superior division of the central retinal artery in the right eye of a 54-year-old man. This looks like a venous occlusion, but the visual field showed a typical inferior loss associated with a superior arterial occlusion. Fig. 6-3, *B* shows the angiogram done at this time. Note particularly the poor filling of the superior nasal vessels. Fig. 6-3, *C* shows the appearance of the fundus 48 hours after the administration of urokinase, and Fig. 6-3, D is the

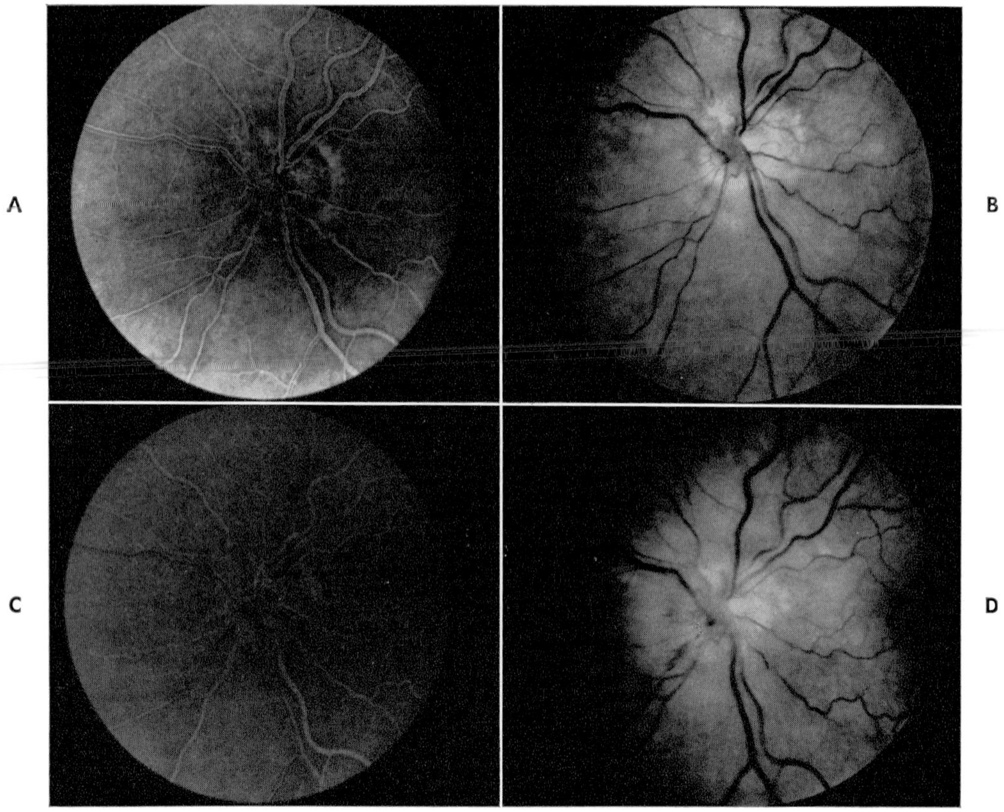

Fig. 6-3. A, Appearance of fundus of patient with an occlusion of the superior division of the central retinal artery. **B,** Fluoroangiogram at initial visit. **C,** Appearance of fundus 48 hours after infusion of urokinase. **D,** Fluoroangiogram 48 hours after administration of urokinase.

angiogram done at this time. Note the improved filling of the superior nasal vessels. Unfortunately, the visual field loss did not improve, but central vision has remained good. A third case of superior arterial occlusion has not fared as well. In spite of treatment the patient's inferior vessels closed later on.

Our one case of central vein occlusion has cleared completely with return of vision to 20/20. In summary, our experience is much too small to allow for definitive conclusions; however, urokinase does seem to hold promise, and it seems to have few toxic side effects. Many more cases must be accumulated before a reliable evaluation can be made.

SUMMARY

As with cerebral occlusions, therapy for arterial and venous occlusions of the retina remains unsatisfactory because of the irreversible changes that take place in a short time. This is obviously as true for the retina as it is for the brain. Anticoagulation by means of heparin and orally administered anticoagulants appears to be a useful treatment and has received acceptance in most centers. The usefulness of plasma expanders and fibrinolytic agents is less solidly documented. At this time our feeling about these agents is as follows:

1. Low molecular weight dextran is of use primarily in the early stages of vascular occlusive disease. Since patients are rarely seen at this time, dextran is not a very useful drug for our purposes. However, it is relatively safe, in spite of occasional reports of renal damage, and its use should be considered in patients who have only one eye and develop a serious occlusion.

2. Fibrinolysin is an effective drug, but its effectiveness appears to be caused by the fact that it contains streptokinase. The latter is a drug that is difficult to manage and can produce many unpleasant side effects. Its usefulness in ophthalmology is not documented, and therefore, it is not advised for treatment at this time in any patient with a retinal vascular occlusion.

3. Urokinase is not as yet available commercially, but it appears to be a safe drug. It deserves a wider clinical trial, and at this time its use should be limited to centers where very careful control is available and where such side effects as increased bleeding may be quickly controlled. Since it is not available, no recommendation need be made on its use at this time.

REFERENCES

1. Zweng, H. C., Little, H. L., and Peabody, R. R.: Laser photocoagulation and retinal angiography, St. Louis, 1969, The C. V. Mosby Co., pp. 112-135.
2. Shoch, D.: Therapy of retinal vascular occlusion. In Leopold, I. H., editor: Symposium on ocular therapy, vol. 4, St. Louis, 1969, The C. V. Mosby Co., p. 61.
3. Mustard, J. F., Rowsell, H. C., and Murphy, E. A.: Thrombosis, Amer. J. Med. Sci. **248**:469, 1964.
4. Jorgensen, L., and Borchgrevink, C. F.: The haemostatic mechanism in patients with haemorrhagic diseases, Acta Path. Microbiol. Scand. **60**:55, 1964.
5. Sawyer, P. N., Brattain, W. H., and Boddy, P. J.: Electrochemical precipitation of human blood cells and its possible relation to intravascular thrombosis, Proc. Nat. Acad. Sci. U.S.A. **51**:428, 1964.
6. Bygdenan, S.: Prevention and therapy of thromboembolic complications with dextran, Progr. Surg. **7**:114, 1969.
7. Gronwall, A., and Ingelman, B.: Dextran as a substitute for plasma, Nature **155**: 45, 1945.
8. Borgstrom, S., Gelin, L. E., and Zederfeldt, B.: The formation of vein thrombi following tissue injury, Acta Clin. Scand. (Suppl. 247), 1959.
9. Rothman, S., Adelson, E., and others: Adsorption of carbon-14 dextran to human blood platelets and red blood cells, in vitro, Vox Sang. **2**:104, 1957.
10. Bloom, W. L., Harmer, D. S., and others: Coating of vascular surfaces and cells: a new concept in prevention of intravascular thrombosis, Proc. Soc. Exp. Biol. Med. **115**:384, 1964.

11. Gilroy, J., Barnhart, M. I., and Meyer, J. S.: Treatment of acute stroke with dextran 40, J. A. M. A. **210**:293, 1969.
12. Antoine, F., Pierre, I., and Martinelle, F.: Le dextran de faible poids moleculaire (rheomacrodex) dans le traitement des troubles circulatiores retiniens, Bull. Soc. Franc. Ophtal. **67**:1156, 1967.
13. Radnot, M., and Follman, P.: Rheomacrodex (dextran) in the treatment of the occlusion of the central retinal vein, Ann. Ophthal. **1**:58, 1969.
14. Daniel, W. J., Mohamed, S. D., and Matheson, N. A.: Treatment of mesenteric embolism with dextran 40, Lancet **1**:567, 1966.
15. Johnson, A. J., and McCarty, W. R.: The lysis of artificially induced intravascular clots in man by intravascular infusions of streptokinase, J. Clin. Invest. **38**:1627, 1959.
16. Alkjaersig, N., Fletcher, A. P., and Sherry, S.: The mechanism of clot dissolution by plasmin, J. Clin. Invest. **38**:1086, 1959.
17. Fletcher, A. P., Alkjaersig, N., and others: Evaluation of human fibrinolysin (Actase), J. A. M. A. **172**:912, 1960.
18. Hecker, S. P., and Zweng, H. C.: Central retinal artery occlusion successfully treated with plasmin, J. A. M. A. **176**:1067, 1961.
19. Jutte, A., and Lemke, L.: Nachweis der Rekanalisation eines Netzhautarterien—verschlusses durch Fluoreszein, Klin. Mbl. Augenheilk. **147**:348, 1965.
19a. Zweng, H. C., Little, H. L., and Peabody, R. R.: Laser photocoagulation and retinal angiography, St. Louis, 1969, The C. V. Mosby Co., p. 124.
20. Fletcher, A. P., Alkjaersig, N., and others: The development of urokinase as a thrombolytic agent: maintenance of a sustained thrombolytic state in man by its intravenous infusion, J. Lab. Clin. Med. **65**:713, 1965.
21. Sautter, R. D., Emanuel, D. A., and others: Urokinase for the treatment of acute pulmonary embolism, J. A. M. A. **202**:215, 1967.
22. Genton, E., and Wolf, P. S.: Urokinase therapy in pulmonary thromboembolism, Amer. Heart J. **76**:628, 1968.

Chapter 7

Immunosuppressive agents in ophthalmology

Vernon G. Wong, M.D.

Physicians are constantly seeking effective treatments for diseases caused by inflammatory or autoimmune mechanisms, or both. Many such conditions are unfortunately common and often run a chronic and disabling course. Although a number of these disorders can be managed successfully with corticosteroids, there are definite therapeutic limitations. Moreover, the success of corticosteroids remains obscure, and a clear understanding of how they improve disease states is still unknown. In a number of inflammatory ocular disorders, the responsiveness to steroid therapy most often is variable and unpredictable. Significantly, the process in many is chronic and so slowly progressive that the hazards of prolonged corticosteroid treatment often outweigh the possible advantages. Because of these uncertainties, it is necessary to search for alternative methods of treatment. The therapeutic agents of choice for diseases caused by inflammatory or immune injury appear to be those that can effectively block the formation of injurious antibodies and immune cells. It seems clear from the available clinical and laboratory observations that a number of the antitumor agents can best fulfill the aforementioned functions.[1-4] Antimetabolites were first introduced as agents in treating immunologic disorders after evidence demonstrated that they were potent inhibitors of antibody synthesis and allograft rejection in experimental situations. The number of such conditions occurring in patients who have been successfully treated with antimetabolites includes systemic lupus erythematosus, autoimmune hemolytic anemia, idiopathic thrombocytopenic purpura, nephrosis, glomerulonephritis, rheumatoid arthritis, psoriasis, ulcerative colitis, plasma cell hepatitis, and many others. The success of experimental and human homograft rejection has been made possible because of the potent antiimmune properties of these agents.[5-13]

At the present time much still remains unknown in the mechanisms of the action of immunosuppressive drugs in the treatment of clinical diseases. Moreover, immunologic lesions are elaborated by complicated mechanisms that can be responsible for the final clinical expression of inflammatory injury. Some of these factors involved are antigen, antibody, sensitized cells, pharmacologic mediators of allergic reactions, complement, and phagocytic and inflammatory cells. Although not all of these mechanisms necessarily participate in a given disorder, chemical therapy of an immunoinflammatory disease must be directed toward their elimination or suppression.

The rationale for administration of antimetabolites in the therapy of ocular inflammatory diseases presupposes that the disease under treatment represents primarily a disorder of immunity. Supportive evidence for this assumption, particularly with reference to endogenous uveitis, has been drawn from several laboratory and clinical studies.[14-24]

Initial effects of these compounds in the treatment of clinical ocular inflammatory syndromes were reported in 1965.[25] Subsequent studies,[26, 27] and the work of others, soon followed, which confirmed the effectiveness of these compounds in refractory cases. Results obtained at the National Institutes of Health in patients treated with azathioprine, cyclophosphamide, or amethopterin showed that over 65% of the treated patients were benefited by the chemotherapy. Corticosteroid therapy failed in each patient because these hormones were ineffective or because severe toxic side effects developed from their use. Consistently favorable responses were seen in those patients with cyclitis and sympathetic ophthalmia. Dramatic resolution of the disease was seen in several patients with scleromalacia perforans, Wegener's granulomatosis, corneal rejection, and pseudotumor of the orbit. In our experience Behçet's and uveal effusion syndromes exhibited little or no improvement.

These results are similar to those reported in the American ophthalmic literature that has been recently surveyed.[28-36] In the published reports, 70% of a total of approximately 100 patients with various refractory inflammatory ocular diseases responded to antimetabolites with complete or partial remission. Among diseases that were also treated were Vogt-Koyanagi syndrome, presumed ocular histoplasmosis, and nonspecific anterior and posterior uveitis. Because of their antiinflammatory effects, these agents were successfully used as adjunctive chemotherapy to post-operative uveitis cases.[27]

Methotrexate, cyclophosphamide, 6-mercaptopurine (6-MP), and azathioprine have been most commonly used in clinical ophthalmology.

The drug doses that have been reported were intravenous methotrexate, 25 mg. per square meter of body surface area every 4 days; intravenous cyclophosphamide, 1 gm. per square meter of body surface area weekly, or 100 mg. by mouth daily; 6-MP, 2.0 to 2.7 mg./kg. of body weight per day, by mouth; and azathioprine, 3 to 5 mg./kg. of body weight per day, by mouth.[37]

Although it has been assumed that antimetabolites exert their beneficial effects by immunosuppression, our experience, as well at that of others, has unfortunately been that there was little correlation between the degree of immunosuppression and clinical response.[27] Furthermore, few patients who failed to respond clinically had notable impairment of their primary and secondary immune responses. That infectious complications have been minimal may be because patients treated were not rendered hypogammaglobulinemic and because they had normal amounts of immunoglobulins that had the usual spectrum of antibacterial and antiviral activities. Moreover, it has been shown that induced leukopenia is not a necessary prerequisite to achieve immunosuppressive clinical effects. It has been our experience that the effectiveness of these agents may lie in their inherent potent antiinflammatory properties rather than in specific suppression of immunoglobulin or alteration of the delayed hypersensitivity mechanisms.

It seems clear from our experience and that of other investigators that immunosuppressive therapy offers definite promise in the treatment of ocular diseases. The major limiting factor, however, in the use of these agents is their toxic side effects. Expert medical management, particularly in the long-term clinical application of these agents, must therefore be used whenever these agents are tried.

In all considerations of clinical use of immunosuppressive drugs, it must be realized that this is a rapidly developing field and much remains to be learned from their application in medicine. Therefore, one can anticipate a future in which effective pharmacology of immunosuppression will permit selective inhibition of unwanted immunologic processes. However, because the type of immunosuppressive effect obtained is presently unpredictable in man, it will be difficult to attempt to define any immunologic diseases until we can determine them in reasonably pathogenetic terms.

REFERENCES

1. Bukantz, S. C., Dammin, G. J., and others: Inhibitory effect of nitrogen mustard (bis B-chloroethylamine) on lesions of experimental serum hypersensitiveness, Proc. Soc. Exp. Biol. Med. **72**:21, 1949.
2. Friedman, R. M., Buckler, C. E., and Baron, S.: The effect of aminomethylpteroylglutamic acid on the development of skin hypersensitivity and on antibody formation in guinea pigs, J. Exp. Med. **114**:173, 1961.

3. Hitchings, G. H., and Elion, G. B.: Chemical suppression of the immune response, Pharmacol. Rev. **15**:365, 1963.
4. Schwartz, R. S.: Immunosuppressive therapy. In Miescher, P., and Grabar, P., editors: Immunopathology, Fifth International Symposium, New York, 1967, Grune & Stratton, Inc., pp. 360-365.
5. Eisen, B., Demis, D. J., and Crosby, W. H.: Thioguanine therapy: systemic lupus erythematosus, atopic dermatitis and other non-malignant diseases, J. A. M. A. **179**:789, 1962.
6. Schwartz, R., and Dameshek, W.: Treatment of autoimmune hemolytic anemia with 6-mercaptopurine and thioguanine, Blood **19**:483, 1962.
7. Wolff, S. M., and Goodman, H. C.: Hypogammaglobulinemia produced by administration of 6-thioguanine to patients with nephrosis, J. Clin. Invest. **41**: 1413, 1962.
8. Black, R. L., O'Brien, W. M., and others: Methotrexate therapy in psoriatic arthritis: a double-blind study on 21 patients, J. A. M. A. **189**:743, 1964.
9. Van Scott, E. J., Auerbach, R., and Weinstein, G. D.: Parenteral methotrexate in psoriasis, Arch. Derm. **89**:550, 1964.
10. Page, A. R., Condie, R. M., and Good, R. A.: Suppression of plasma cell hepatitis with 6-mercaptopurine, Amer. J. Med. **36**:200, 1964.
11. Swanson, M., and Schwartz, R. S.: Immunosuppressive therapy: relation between immunological competence and clinical responsiveness, New Eng. J. Med. **277**:163, 1967.
12. Murray, J. E., Wilson, R. E., and others: Five years' experience in renal transplantation with immunosuppressive drugs: survival, function, complications, and the role of lymphocyte depletion by thoracic duct fistula, Ann. Surg. **168**:416, 1968.
13. Barnard, C. N.: A human cardiac transplant: an interim report of a successful operation performed at Groote Schuur Hospital, Cape Town, S. Afr. Med. J. **41**: 1271, 1967.
14. Collins, R. C.: Experimental studies on sympathetic ophthalmia, Amer. J. Ophthal. **32**:1687, 1949.
15. Suie, T., and Dodd, M. C.: An immunologic study of rabbits sensitized with homologuous uveal tissue, Amer. J. Ophthal. **39**:377, 1955.
16. Miescher, A.: Experimentelle untersuchunger zur pathogenese der sympathischen opthalmie, Ophthalmologica **130**:128, 1955.
17. Aronson, S. B.: The homo-immune uveitises in the guinea pig, Ann. N. Y. Acad. Sci. **124**:365, 1965.
18. Wacker, W. B., and Lipton, M. M.: Experimental allergic uveitis: homologous retina as uveitogenic antigen, Nature **206**:253, 1965.
19. Wacker, W. B., Lipton, M. M., and Ougchua, F. E.: Antibody production in the guinea pig to homologous uvea, Proc. Soc. Exp. Biol. Med. **117**:150, 1964.
20. Woods, A. C.: Immune reactions following injuries to the uveal tract, J. A. M. A. **77**:1317, 1921.
21. Hallett, J. W., and others: Auto-immune complement fixation test in endogenous uveitis, Arch. Ophthal. **68**:168, 1962.
22. Remky, H.: Auto-anticorps facteurs endogenes de l'iritis, Soc. Franc. Ophtal. **78**:401, 1965.
23. Aronson, S. B., Schnellmann, D. L., and Yamamoto, E. A.: Uveal autoantibody in ocular disease, J. A. M. A. **196**:225, 1966.
24. Wirostko, E., and Halbert, S. P.: Suppression of allergic uveitis by 6-mercaptopurine, J. Exp. Med. **116**:653, 1962.
25. Wong, V. G., and Hersh, E. M.: Methotrexate in the therapy of cyclitis, Trans. Amer. Acad. Ophthal. Otolaryng. **69**:279, 1965.
26. Wong, V. G., Hersh, E. M., and McMaster, P. R. B.: Treatment of a presumed case of sympathetic ophthalmia with methotrexate, Arch. Ophthal. **76**:66, 1966.

27. Wong, V. G.: Immunosuppressive therapy of ocular inflammatory diseases, Arch. Ophthal. **81**:628, 1969.
28. Newell, F. W., Krill, A. E., and Thomson, A.: The treatment of uveitis with six-mercaptopurine, Amer. J. Ophthal. **61**:1250, 1966.
29. Bignell, J. L., and Mackay, I.: Chronic uveitis as an auto-immune disease: the result of treatment with azathioprine (Imuran). Presented at XX Concilium Ophthalmologicum Germania. International Congress Series N., **146**:645, 1966.
30. Newel, F. W., and Krill, A. E.: Treatment of uveitis with azathioprine (Imuran), Trans. Ophthal. Soc. U. K. **87**:499, 1967.
31. Mackay, I. R., and Bignell, J. L.: Prevention of corneal-graft failure with the immunosuppressive drug azathioprine, Lancet **2**:479, 1967.
32. Gills, J. P.: Combined medical and surgical therapy for complicated cases of peripheral uveitis, Arch. Ophthal. **79**:723, 1968.
33. Moore, C. E.: Sympathetic ophthalmitis treated with azathioprine, Brit. J. Ophthal. **52**:688, 1968.
34. Mathews, J. D., Crawford, B. A., and others: Azathioprine in active chronic iridocyclitis, Brit. J. Ophthal. **53**:327, 1969.
35. Lazar, M., Weiner, M. J., and Leopold, I. H.: Treatment of uveitis with methotrexate, Amer. J. Ophthal. **67**:383, 1969.
36. Buckley, S. E., and Gills, J. P., Jr.: Cyclophosphamide therapy of peripheral uveitis, Arch. Intern. Med. **124**:29, 1969.
37. Wong, V. G.: Immunosuppressive agents in ophthalmology, Survey Ophthal. **13**:290, 1969.

Chapter 8

Management and complications of systemic corticosteroid therapy

John E. Harris, M.D., Ph.D.

The corticosteroids have come to be widely used in ophthalmology since the introduction of cortisone and adrenocorticotropic hormone (ACTH) in 1949. Our concern here is not so much with the type of ocular disease most likely to respond to corticosteroids but rather with the management of the patient while he is on systemic therapy.

There is probably little indication for the use of ACTH in ocular disease. It has been used in the treatment of multiple sclerosis,[1, 2] particularly in the acute stage. The androgenic steroids, released along with cortisol when the adrenals are stimulated, are felt to minimize the myopathic effect of the glucocorticosteroids.[3] In a controlled study, ACTH was found to be of value in the treatment of acute retrobulbar neuritis.[4] The patients were given 40 units of ACTH gel intramuscularly for a total of 30 days.

In Table 8-1 are listed some of the more commonly used corticosteroids that are now available. The relative antiinflammatory potency and sodium-retaining activity of the various corticosteroids, using hydrocortisone or cortisol as the reference drug, are indicated in Table 8-2. It should be emphasized that the antiinflammatory data have been drawn from a number of sources, particularly animal studies. While they are generally in the realm of reality, any specific transfer from one corticosteroid to another on the dosage ratio shown may not produce the expected effect. In the final analysis the comparative antiinflammatory potency of the various analogs has not been determined with precision

Table 8-1. Trade names and tablet size of more commonly used corticosteroids

Generic name	*Tablet size (mg.)*	*Trade name*
Prednisone	1, 2.5, 5	Deltasone, Deltra, Meticorten, Paracort
Prednisolone	1, 2.5, 5	Co-Hydeltra Deltra cortef, Hydeltra, Meticortelone, Paracortol, Sterane, Sterolone
Triamcinolone	1, 2, 4, 8, 16	Aristocort, Kenacort
Methylprednisolone	2, 4, 16	Medrol
Paramethasone	1, 2	Haldrone
Dexamethasone	0.25, 0.5, 0.75, 1.5	Decadron, Deronil, Dexameth, Gammacorten, Hexadrol
Betamethasone	0.6	Celestone

Table 8-2. Comparison of antiinflammatory and mineralocorticoid activity of some corticosteroids

Compound	*Relative antiinflammatory potency*	*Relative sodium-retaining potency*
Cortisol	1	1
Prednisolone	4	0.8
Prednisone	4	0.8
Methylprednisolone	5	0
Triamcinolone	5	0
Paramethasone	10	0
Betamethasone	25	0
Dexamethasone	25	0

in human beings. There is no good evidence that, given in full therapeutic dose, the antiinflammatory activity of one particular corticosteroid is better than another. It is true that the in vivo half-life of some drugs, such as dexamethasone, is longer than that of others, such as prednisolone,[5] but this is not an important factor in making a choice in the drug to be used. The major considerations in the choice of the drug are the side effects and the cost to the patient.

The principal benefit resulting from the synthesis of the newer corticosteroid analogs (initially prednisone and prednisolone, followed by others) was a reduction in the sodium-retaining potential. Although prednisone and prednisolone cause sodium retention, this is not a problem in most patients who are taking these drugs. If one adds the cost factor to the consideration, prednisone is clearly the drug of choice. In Table 8-3 are listed the relative costs of some of the corticosteroids based on the charges to the University of Minnesota Hospital Pharmacy. Since prednisolone has essentially the same activity as prednisone (indeed prednisone is probably converted to prednisolone in vivo[5]) and yet costs about 2½ times as much, there is no indication for its use.

Table 8-3. Some relative costs*

Compound	*Cost (in dollars)*
Prednisone (5 mg.)	0.95
Prednisolone (5 mg.)	2.40
Triamcinolone (4 mg.)	14.20
Methylprednisolone (4 mg.)	14.50
Paramethasone (2 mg.)	16.00
Dexamethasone (0.75 mg.)	6.50
Betamethasone (0.6 mg.)	16.00

*Based on University of Minnesota Hospital Pharmacy.

Table 8-4. Usual starting therapeutic dosage per day

Compound	*Dosage (mg.)*
Prednisolone (5 mg.)	40 to 60
Prednisone (5 mg.)	40 to 60
Methylprednisolone (4 mg.)	32 to 48
Triamcinolone (4 mg.)	32 to 48
Paramethasone (2 mg.)	16 to 24
Dexamethasone (0.75 mg.)	6 to 9
Bethamethasone (0.6 mg.)	4.8 to 7.2

If sodium retention becomes a factor, switching to dexamethasone is indicated. It costs considerably more than prednisone, but not as much as some of the others. An equally good alternative is to use some naturetic agent, such as one of the thiazides. Triamcinolone has one advantage in this regard in that it is often a naturetic agent. The drugs of choice therefore are prednisone, dexamethasone, and triamcinolone, in that order. Dexamethasone stimulates the appetite considerably, and excessive weight gain may result.[6] This may be an advantage in certain cases but a disadvantage in others. Triamcinolone, on the other hand, depresses the appetite and is the drug of choice when sodium retention and increased appetite present problems. Dexamethasone tends to make the patient euphoric, while triamcinolone acts as a mood depressant.[6]

Table 8-4 summarizes the usual starting therapeutic dosage in ophthalmic disease. For the most part ophthalmic problems require short term therapy, that is, up to 2 to 3 months of therapy, as distinguished from the treatment of chronic diseases, such as asthma, rheumatoid arthritis, nephrotic syndrome, and so on. Thus, it is sound to start off with a relatively high dose to determine whether the process being treated will respond. The alternative, starting with a small dose and gradually increasing it, results in a loss of valuable days of therapy and makes it more difficult to determine whether the inflammatory process is responding to the corticosteroid. In the more chronic ocular diseases this is often difficult to determine, but high dosages can generally be given for a few weeks without great danger, and determinations of the efficacy of the corticosteroid therapy can be made. If response is not evident within a few days, increasing the dosage of prednisone to 100 mg. or dexamethasone to 15 mg. per day or more is not out of order.

Several regimens of therapy have been advocated as a means of reducing the known undesirable metabolic effects of the drugs. (There is no particular advantage of parenteral therapy, so the corticosteroids should be given orally.) Of the various schedules employed, there are three that are considered best. The first is the divided daily dose, usually four times a day. This will provide full therapeutic response but may also result in maximum side effects. The single daily dosage has been advocated by Grant and associates.[7] They have produced evidence that it provides some protection to the hypothalamic–pituitary–adrenal gland axis. The drug should be taken in the morning, since this is the time when the pituitary is least likely to be depressed. An every-other-day dosage has been advocated by Harter and associates.[8] To determine the total dosage needed it is recommended that the patient be started on a divided daily dosage. When the amount needed to control the disease has been established, the total 48-hour dosage is given every other morning. The alternate-day dosage has the advantage of minimizing somewhat the unwanted side effects of the drugs, particularly since it minimizes, although it does not prevent, the depression of the hypothalamic–pituitary–adrenal gland axis.[9] This makes it possible, therefore, to stop the drug fairly abruptly if necessary. The main disadvantage of the alternate-day dosage is that the disease process may not be controlled. If it is anticipated that therapy will be relatively short, such as a period of a few months, the single daily dose is preferred. If the therapy will be prolonged, the alternate-day therapy is advisable. It is always possible to switch from one form of therapy to the other. For the most part in ophthalmic diseases a single daily dose is the preferable treatment.

Once therapy has been demonstrated to be effective, it is imperative to reduce the dosage as soon as possible. There is no good rule of thumb that can apply in all cases. In some instances too rapid a reduction of steroid therapy may cause a return of an inflammatory process. Where concern is simply management of the disease process and the drug being employed is prednisone, reduction in increments of 10 mg. per day once or twice weekly can be made until 20 mg. is reached. Thereafter reduction in the amount of 1 to 5 mg. per day is recommended, the level depending on the duration of therapy and the intensity of the disease. Five mg. of prednisone (and appropriate doses of other drugs) is the equivalent to the output by the adrenal gland of cortisol, and once this dose has been reached, therapy should be stopped if possible.

After prolonged therapy, when the depression of hypothalamic–pituitary–adrenal axis is a concern, cutting off from the maintenance level may become a difficult matter. In such instances Thorn[3] recommends switching to an equivalent dose of dexamethasone, while measuring the urinary 17-hydroxysteroid excretion and the effect thereon of ACTH administration.

While there are some claims in the literature that if one corticosteroid fails to produce an adequate therapeutic response another one will, there appears to be no sound evidence for this. Thus, once the corticosteroid of choice has been given adequate therapeutic trial with no evident clinical benefit, switching to another probably will produce equally disappointing results.

Use of corticosteroids is complicated by certain side effects that are hazardous in various degrees to the patient. A careful history is imperative, and in certain cases special tests may be advisable. From the medical standpoint, among the more benign side effects that may cause the patient concern are the cushionoid characteristics of moon face, acne, striae, hirsutism, and so on.

Among the more serious complications in the use of corticosteroids is the development of a peptic ulcer. The exact mechanisms by which the corticosteroids induce such an ulcer are not known. A patient with past or present evidence of a peptic ulcer diathesis is prone to have his symptoms increased. An upper G.I. series is advised in these patients. The presence of a healed or even an active ulcer does not preclude the use of corticosteroids when adequate care is taken. This would include the use of an ulcer diet, antacids, and examination of the stool for occult blood. In the absence of any history of peptic ulcer an antacid is probably still advisable. It is our pratice to prescribe routinely an antacid for a patient who has no history of peptic ulcer diathesis.

One should always be on the alert for the unmasking of a latent diabetic. A family history of diabetes should make one wary. When diabetes develops it will generally appear early in the course of therapy. It is controlled by the usual methods. Some patients may become insulin dependent, while others can be controlled with oral hypoglycemic agents. As the patient is taken off his corticosteroid therapy, the need for insulin or other hypoglycemic agents is reduced and may disappear. The known diabetic will usually have an increased requirement for hypoglycemic agents. However, we have observed an instance where the need for oral hypoglycemic agents was reduced when the patient was placed on corticosteroid therapy. This may be related to the fact that the amount of insulin released by these agents increases during the therapy.[10]

Osteoporosis is another complication that is likely to be encountered, particularly in older individuals and especially in postmenopausal females. Before starting such an individual on corticosteroids, x-rays of the spine and pelvis are advisable. Patients with demonstrable and particularly severe osteoporosis represent a definite risk, particularly in long-term therapy. However, corticosteroid therapy can be employed if it is felt to be necessary. Adequate protein intake is advised as well as added calcium intake in the form of calcium lactate or gluconate. The usual dosage of calcium lactate is two teaspoonsful a day. An androgenic agent may also be added to the regimen. The benefits of these measures, however, are probably slight.

When the patient has a history of tuberculosis or other chronic infection, the use of corticosteroids should be approached warily, since they may cause an exacerbation of the disease. A chest film is necessary in the patient with healed tuberculosis. Three hundred mg. of isoniazid (INH) per day is recommended while any such patient is on corticosteroids. We routinely employ this in patients with sarcoidosis, since it is often difficult to rule out tuberculosis in these instances. Similarly, the development of an intercurrent infection such as pneumonia, which may be masked by the corticosteroids, must be watched for and treated.

In patients with hypertension or low cardiac reserve, corticosteroids may cause a retention of fluid. In these instances it is best to utilize the regimen suggested previously, that is, switch to dexamethasone or triamcinolone. The corticosteroids are also kaluretic. This is particularly true of prednisone. In the event that the corticosteroids are employed with other drugs that are kaluretics, an additive effect may result. In such cases serum potassium may not adequately reflect the total potassium depletion in the body. Hence, patients on combinations of drugs such as the thiazides or carbonic anhydrase inhibitors and corticosteroids should have potassium supplementation, particularly if they are taking digitalis or one of its derivatives. This is best supplied in the form of natural foods. Two 8-ounce glasses of orange juice a day provide somewhat in excess of 20 mEq. of potassium, which is considered adequate. Potassium supplements are also available.

The use of corticosteroids is accompanied in some patients by profound psychologic changes that may actually lead to a psychosis. It is difficult to predict which patients might have complications, but the complications may be of sufficient severity to cause cessation of therapy.

In patients who have been on corticosteroids in the past, the response to stress such as surgery may lead to some form of adrenal shock. The response to such stress can be tested for;[11] but in actual practice fortifying the patient with corticosteroids prior to and after surgery is all that is necessary. It can be in the form of 100 mg. hydrocortisone succinate given intravenously at the time of surgery. In addition, 200 mg.

cortisone acetate given intramuscularly 12 and 2 hours prior to the surgery may be advisable.

The particular problem of corticosteroid-induced retardation of statural growth in children should be mentioned. Such retardation is not of significance in short-term (2 to 3 months) therapy but is of great importance in long term therapy.[12, 13, 14] When long-term therapy is undertaken in children, alternate-day therapy employing a single dose every other morning is advised, since it has been shown that corticosteroids so administered do not depress statural growth.[15, 16]

REFERENCES

1. Rinne, U. K., Sonninen, V., and Tuovinen, T.: Corticotrophin treatment in multiple sclerosis, Acta Neurol. Scand. **44**:207, 1968.
2. Rose, A. S., Kuzma, J. W., and others: Cooperative study in the evaluation of therapy in multiple sclerosis; ACTH vs. placebo in acute exacerbations, Neurology **20**:1, 1970.
3. Thorn, G. W.: Clinical considerations in the use of corticosteroids, New Eng. J. Med. **274**:775, 1966.
4. Rawson, M. D., Liversedge, L. A., and Goldfarb, G.: Treatment of acute retrobulbar neuritis with corticotrophin, Lancet **11**:1044, 1966.
5. Peterson, R. E.: Metabolism of adrenocorticosteroids in man, Ann. N. Y. Acad. Sci. **82**:846, 1959.
6. Rothermich, N. O.: An updated look at antirheumatic drugs, Med. Clin. N. Amer. **51**:1213, 1967.
7. Grant, S. D., Forsham, P. H., and DiRaimondo, V. C.: Suppression of 17-hydroxycorticosteroids in plasma and urine by single and divided doses of triamcinolone, New Eng. J. Med. **273**:1115, 1965.
8. Harter, J. G., Reddy, W. J., and Thorn, G. W.: Studies on an intermittent corticosteroid dosage regimen, New Eng. J. Med. **269**:591, 1963.
9. Siegel, S. C., Heimlich, E. M., and others: Effects of alternate-day steroid therapy in asthmatic children, J. Allergy **36**:209, 1965 (Abstract).
10. Perley, M., and Kipnis, D. M.: Effect of glucocorticoids on plasma insulin, New Eng. J. Med. **274**:1238, 1966.
11. Jasani, M. K., Freeman, P. A., and others: Studies of the rise in plasma 11-hydroxycorticosteroids (11-OHCS) in corticosteroid-treated patients with rheumatoid arthritis during surgery: correlations with the functional integrity of the hypothalamopituitary-adrenal axis, Quart. J. Med. **147**:407, 1968.
12. Blodgett, F. M., Burgin, L., and others: Effects of prolonged cortisone therapy on the statural growth, skeletal maturation and metabolic status of children, New Eng. J. Med. **254**:636, 1956.
13. Van Metre, T. E., and Pinkerton, H. L.: Growth suppression in asthmatic children receiving prolonged therapy with prednisolone and methyl prednisolone, J. Allergy **30**:103, 1959.
14. Falliers, C. J., Tan, L. S., and others: Childhood asthma and steroid therapy as influences on growth, Amer. J. Dis. Child. **105**:127, 1963.
15. Soyka, L. F.: Treatment of nephrotic syndrome in childhood, Amer. J. Dis. Child. **113**:693, 1967.
16. Johnston, J. A., Manson, G., and others: Intermittent steroid therapy in nephrosis, Amer. J. Dis. Child. **114**:288, 1967.

Chapter 9

Corticosteroids in infectious corneal disease

Samuel B. Aronson, M.D., and Thomas E. Moore, Jr., M.D.

The utilization of corticosteroids in corneal inflammation has provoked considerable controversy since the introduction of these agents more than 20 years ago. Some initial reports indicated that corticosteroids offered a marvelous therapeutic spectrum in keratitis of various causes.[1, 2] This position was rapidly succeeded by a negative swing of the pendulum; corticosteroids became suspected of leading to most of the severe corneal complications that the ophthalmologist encountered.[3, 4] As we enter the new decade, it appears that the pendulum has swung to a more tolerant position. In general, when the causative agent in an infectious disease process can be controlled, the ravages of the inflammatory process can be prevented or ameliorated markedly by corticosteroid therapy.

Our use of corticosteroids is based on the observation that inflammation can destroy useful function more easily and rapidly in the eye than in other systemic organs, which seem able to endure considerable inflammation without functional compromise. The cornea best exemplifies this unique susceptibility of ocular tissue: even minimal scarring seriously impairs vision. Thus, the preservation of corneal structure must be a prime objective in achieving a satisfactory therapeutic result. This chapter reports our most recent experiences with combined corticosteroid and antimicrobial therapy in infectious keratitis.

From the Eye Research Laboratories, Department of Ophthalmology, and the Clinical Laboratories, San Francisco General Hospital, University of California. This study was supported in part by U. S. Public Health Service research grants EY 00246 and EY 00408; Dr. Aronson is the recipient of the U. S. Public Health Service Research Career Development Award K3 NB 31, 653.

METHODS OF PROCEDURE

Selection of patients

Patients with complaints or primary signs of corneal infectious disease came to the emergency ward or outpatient clinic at San Francisco General Hospital (S.F.G.H.); some were referred in private consultations to one of us. On presentation, each patient was examined by both of us, and severity of corneal disease was classified according to a clinicomorphologic gradient. If disparity in classification occurred we discussed our observations until agreement was achieved.

Patients included in this study demonstrated infiltrative corneal disease, which can be divided into central stromal keratitis[5] and peripheral infiltrative disease.[6] The designation of these inflammations as infiltrative disease is based upon early clinical signs that appeared as infiltrates of polymorphonuclear leukocytes (PMN) in the central or peripheral corneal stroma. We believe that this reaction represents chemotaxis and phagocytosis by the PMN in response to toxic or immune stimuli utilizing the complement-binding (acute inflammatory) pathway.[7] Our clinicomorphologic classification encompasses a description of epithelial, stromal, and endothelial clinical changes. In central stromal keratitis any lesion that demonstrates stromal infiltrate is treated with combined corticosteroid therapy. Generally speaking, permanent structural change occurs when (1) central corneal endothelium is destroyed by the inflammatory process or (2) severe corneal neovascularization leads to dense central leukoma formation. Specific infectious etiologic agents in this group are herpes simplex virus, herpes zoster virus, *Staphylococcus aureus, Pneumococcus, Pseudomonas, Moraxella*, β-hemolytic *Streptococcus*, and the fungi *Candida albicans* and *Aspergillus*.

Peripheral infiltrative lesions may occur as part of an acute conjunctivitis syndrome or as a relatively isolated finding secondary to a zone of limbal hyperemia.[6] In the acute (initial) form lesions may occur as isolated foci of PMN in the anterior peripheral corneal stroma, with or without superficial corneal neovascularization, or they may spread diffusely throughout the anterior corneal stroma as in epidemic keratoconjunctivitis (EKC). More chronic inflammation exhibits pannus formation (a superficial, subepithelial, fibrovascular membrane) in various stages of progression toward the central cornea. During active inflammation the pannus frequently demonstrates a zone of coalesced infiltrate along the corneal margin. Specific infectious agents that compose the acute (initial) microbial group are *Staphylococcus aureus* or *epidermidis*, trachoma–inclusion conjunctivitis (TRIC) agent, adenovirus (type 8, EKC), and cases identified during a mixed strain adenovirus epidemic. *Staphylococcus aureus* infections comprise the chronic microbial pannus group in this study.

Peripheral corneal ischemia occurs secondarily to severe peripheral infiltrative syndromes. The morphologic sequence shows severe ischemic edema following infiltrate formation. This rapidly progresses to breakdown and sloughing of the anterior stroma, presenting at this stage as a typical peripheral corneal ulcer. We have identified this change in peripheral herpes simplex virus, *Pseudomonas*, *Gonococcus*, and *Staphylococcus aureus* infections.

The etiologic agent was diagnosed by culture or typical clinical picture. Bacterial and fungal agents were identified by conjunctival or corneal culture (conjunctival and corneal cases). The former were plated on blood and chocolate agar plates (bacteria) or Sabouraud's media (fungi). The latter were first injected into a brain infusion medium for 24 hours, then subplated.* TRIC agent was identified as an intracytoplasmic inclusion by Giemsa stain. Herpes simplex infection was identified by observation of an epithelial dendrite. Herpes zoster infection was identified by its peculiar dermatomal pattern.

Immunologic evaluation

All patients were evaluated immunologically prior to combined corticosteroid therapy.[5-9] Immunologic tests included protein electrophoresis, qualitative immunoelectrophoresis, quantitative immunoglobulins, and B_1C. If a patient demonstrated questionable immunologic incompetence (IgG $>$ 2 SD below normal), he was treated with corticosteroid only after cultures were negative. When IgM was diminished (IgM $>$ 1 SD below mean), the patient was started on combined therapy and was observed closely throughout active therapy.

Patterns of therapy

All patients with central infiltrative keratitis were treated topically with the appropriate antibiotic[5] and corticosteroid (prednisolone acetate 1% suspension, one drop hourly between 6:00 A.M. and 10:00 P.M.). If the reaction was severely destructive, corticosteroid (dexamethasone [Decadron] 4 mg./ml., 0.8 ml., lidocaine [Xylocaine] 2%, 0.2 ml.) was injected subconjunctivally four times a day until inflammatory severity subsided. Corticosteroid was rapidly tapered and discontinued when corneal infiltrates had resolved. Topical antibiotic therapy was matched to corticosteroid dosage, that is, one drop hourly between 6:00 A.M. and 10:00 P.M. Antibiotics most frequently used included neomycin (Neosporin) for *Staphylococcus*, tetracycline for β-hemolytic *Streptococcus* and *Gonococcus*, and chloramphenicol (Chloromycetin) for the diphtheroid cases. IDU was used in matched dosage in cases of herpes simplex. Both fungus

*Cultures were evaluated by W. K. Hadley, M.D., Ph.D., Chief of Bacteriology, Clinical Laboratories, San Francisco General Hospital.

cases were treated with topical amphotericin B and nystatin preparations prior to corticosteroid therapy. No antimicrobial agent was used in herpes zoster cases. Systemic antibiotics were included on evidence of severe lid or orbital involvement or evidence of a systemic infection. Systemic antibiotics included orally or intramuscularly administered penicillin G in β hemolytic *Streptococcus* and *Gonococcus* cases and penicillin G or ampicillin in the *Staphylococcus* cases.

Peripheral infiltrative corneal cases were treated with hourly topical corticosteroid therapy and antibiotics in the regimen described for central stromal keratitis. These patients demonstrated rapid clearing, usually requiring no more than 1 week of therapy.

Patients with identified TRIC agent were examined for concomitant involvement of genitalia. When involvement was present, they were treated with systemic tetracycline, 1,000 mg. per day for 3 weeks, in addition to topical tetracycline therapy. Chronic pannus formation was treated periodically with combined topical therapy. Therapy in peripheral ischemic syndromes is characterized by the addition of subconjunctival heparin to the topical combined corticosteroid-antimicrobial regimen used in infectious peripheral infiltrative disease. Heparin sodium dosage is 300 μ heparin every second day for five doses (heparin sodium 0.3 ml. of 1,000 μ/ml. solution, 0.2 ml. of 2% lidocaine, and 0.5 ml. of sodium chloride). This dilution is injected adjacent to the area of ischemia. Neovascularization and filling-in of the bed of the lesion will occur in the course of the therapeutic regimen.

Long-term patient follow-up

We have attempted to follow all patients on an outpatient basis at routine intervals. Yearly clinicomorphologic reclassification, as well as microbial and immunologic studies, has been performed. Only patients followed for longer than 1 year have been considered in determination of recurrence rates.

RESULTS

Infiltrative corneal disease

Our experience in acute central stromal keratitis has been reported previously;[5] this series has been updated in Table 9-1. At present we have treated 146 patients with acute corneal inflammation, 143 of whom have achieved inflammatory inactivation while on combined corticosteroid therapy. Sixty-four (44%) of these achieved visual acuity (VA) > 20/40 without a subsequent penetrating keratoplasty. Seventy-two of the remaining patients subsequently required keratoplasty (Table 9-2); 52 patients (70%) achieved successful grafts, 44 patients (60%) achieved VA of > 20/40. In all, 108 of 145 patients (74%) achieved central VA of > 20/40.

Table 9-1. Results of combined therapy in acute central stromal keratitis

Etiologic agent	*Total patients*	*Improved with treatment*		*VA > 20/40*	
		Number	*Percent*	*Number*	*Percent*
Herpes simplex	81	79	98	38	47
Herpes zoster	19	19	100	12	63
*Staphylococcus aureus**	16	16	100	6	38
*Pneumococcus**	9	9	100	2	22
*Pseudomonas**	10	9	90	2	20
*Moraxella**	6	6	100	2	33
β-hemolytic *Streptococcus**	3	3	100	2	66
Fungi	2	2	100	0	0
Total	146	143	98	64	44

*Includes 29 primary bacterial infections and 15 that occurred secondarily in keratoplasties.

Table 9-2. Results of combined therapy with keratoplasty in acute central stromal keratitis*

Etiologic diagnosis	*Total cases*	*Successful grafts*		*VA > 20/40*	
		Number	*Percent*	*Number*	*Percent*
Herpes simplex	40	27	68	24	60
Herpes zoster	7	7	100	5	71
Bacteria†	25	17	64	14	56
Fungi	2	1	50	1	50
Total	74	52	70	44	60

*Follow-up > 1 year.
†Includes both preoperative diagnosis and postkeratoplasty infections.

Table 9-3. Recurrent inflammation following combined therapy in infectious central stromal keratitis

Diagnostic group	*Patients followed*	*Recurrenct inflammation*	
		Number	*Percent*
Herpes simplex	32	20	63
Herpes zoster	8	4	50
Bacteria	8	7	87
Total	48	31	65

In general there was no specific relationship between visual outcome and any given etiologic agent. The determining factor in attaining a good visual result without a subsequent keratoplasty was the severity of corneal involvement at the time of initial presentation. If the visual axis was severely involved, the patient was likely to require subsequent surgery.[6]

The rate of recurrent inflammation in unoperated patients during

Table 9-4. Recurrent inflammation following penetrating keratoplasty in infectious central stromal keratitis

Diagnostic group	Patients followed	Recurrent inflammation Number	Recurrent inflammation Percent
Herpes simplex	33	8	24
Herpes zoster	6	1	16
Bacterial keratitis*	6	1	16
Fungi	1	0	0
Total	46	10	22

*Only preoperative diagnosis included.

Table 9-5. Correlation between recurrent inflammation and socioeconomic status

Socioeconomic group	Total patients	Recurrent inflammation Number	Recurrent inflammation Percent
Central stromal keratitis			
S.F.G.H.	25	23	92
Private	23	8	35
Penetrating keratoplasty			
S.F.G.H.	23	20	87
Private	88	19	22

the first year following combined therapy is presented in Table 9-3. Sixty-five percent experienced some degree of recurrent corneal inflammation. This percentage proved to be slightly higher in herpes simplex keratitis than in other diagnostic categories. Three patients with herpes simplex infection, two patients with herpes zoster infection, and two patients with bacterial infection required penetrating keratoplasty to improve vision after inactivation of the recurrent attack.

The overall rate of inflammatory recurrence, 22%, was appreciably lower following penetrating keratoplasty (Table 9-4). Herpes simplex infection recurrence rates declined dramatically from 63% to 24%. In general terms, the severity of corneal structural alteration is diminished following penetrating keratoplasty. Recently, while reviewing recurrence figures we have noted that the incidence of recurrent corneal inflammation is appreciably higher in indigent patients than in private patients (Table 9-5). This proved to be true for both unoperated and operated patient series. It is particularly interesting to note in nonoperated herpes simplex infection cases that 92% of indigent patients (at the S.F.G.H.) demonstrated recurrence as compared to 35% of private patients.

Table 9-6 presents the efficacy of combined corticosteroid therapy in

Table 9-6. Results of combined therapy in acute infectious peripheral corneal disease

Disease group	*Number of patients*	*Number of eyes*	*Improved (eyes)*	
			Number	*Percent*
Acute microbial				
Bacterial	22	34	31	91
Viral	10	16	15	48
Total	32	50	46	92
Chronic microbial				
Bacterial	8	15	14	93
Viral	—	—	—	—
Overall total	40	65	60	92

Table 9-7. Recurrence of acute infectious peripheral corneal disease

Disease group	*Number of patients*	*Number of eyes*	*Recurrence*	
			Number	*Percent*
Acute microbial				
Bacterial	14	22	3	14
Viral	7	12	0	0
Total	21	34		10
Chronic microbial				
Bacterial	6	12	11	92
Viral	—	—	—	—

peripheral infiltrative disease. In both acute and chronic lesions combined corticosteroid therapy was effective in every case, providing the diagnosis of pathogenesis of the peripheral lesion was accurate. (Confusion with secondary microbial ischemic necrosis may occur; in this case antibiotic corticosteroid therapy should be combined with heparin.) Similarly, therapy must be continued until the stimulating agent is under control. If stopped too soon, inflammatory activity will recur; for example, three patients with adenovirus infection (EKC) demonstrated reappearance of corneal infiltrates following discontinuation of corticosteroid therapy. These infiltrates rapidly disappeared when administration of corticosteroids was resumed.

The recurrence rate of peripheral infiltrative disease is directly related to the degree of permanent structural change in the peripheral cornea and limbus (Table 9-7). The acute microbial group, in which minimal structural change occurred, showed only one recurrent case during the 1-year follow-up period. (This recurrence was a *Staphylococcus* infection in an individual who had presented initially with a TRIC

Table 9-8. Combined corticosteroid-heparin therapy in infectious peripheral ischemic syndromes

Etiologic agent	*Number of patients*	*Number of eyes*	*Improved*	
			Number	*Percent*
Herpes simplex	3	3	3	100
Pseudomonas	1	2	2	100
Gonococcus	2	2	2	100
Staphylococcus aureus	2	2	2	100
Total	8	9	9	100

infection.) However, every case with chronic change (pannus) demonstrated multiple recurrences during the follow-up year. In two staphylococcal cases, infiltrates could be controlled only by continuing active combined neomycin and corticosteroid therapy.

Ischemia of the peripheral cornea secondary to severe microbial infections presented a unique therapeutic situation. These cases started as peripheral infiltrative lesions but soon demonstrated evidence of ischemia, that is, some degree of dissolution of the peripheral corneal stroma. When infiltrative diseases are appropriately treated (heparin, corticosteroid, and antimicrobial therapy), an excellent prognosis can be achieved (Table 9-8).

DISCUSSION

Corticosteroid-antimicrobial therapy in acute infectious corneal infiltrative diseases

In the course of these studies, 178 patients (196 eyes) have received high dosage, topical or subconjunctival, corticosteroid therapy in combination with appropriate antimicrobial therapy. Of this group, 189 eyes (> 95%) improved dramatically. Three patients in the central stromal keratitis series showed complications, which, once recognized, were readily controlled.[5, 6]

The rationale behind corticosteroid therapy in infectious ocular disease is suppression of the overall inflammatory reaction, particularly the PMN component, which in turn limits destruction of ocular tissue. The PMN is the principal carrier of hydrolytic enzymes that are probably responsible for most parenchymal destruction.[10, 11] By interrupting this reaction, corticosteriod therapy serves to reduce the severity of the inflammatory response. We believe that such changes as corneal stromal scarring and neovascularization, as well as secondary endothelial decompensation, can be avoided if corticosteroids are introduced early enough in the course of the infectious disease process.

As noted earlier in this chapter, corticosteroid therapy is administered by topical application or subconjunctival injection, principally because the facility of these routes in attaining optimal therapy has been confirmed by a number of experiments.[12-15] These routes also preclude or diminish markedly the side effects of systemic administration. If systemic therapy is necessary we believe that it should be started at very high levels and continued no longer than 10 to 14 days.

The effect of corticosteroid therapy on the infectious agents merits some consideration. In general, corticosteroid therapy alone seems to encourage microbial proliferation, that is, proliferation of herpes simplex virus,[16-18] *Pseudomonas,*[19] and the tubercle bacillus.[20, 21] The mechanism of this enhanced proliferation has not been determined. Whether the mechanism is a direct effect of corticosteroid therapy on the agent's replication[22] or an indirect effect by interfering with the host response,[23, 24] remains speculative. More pertinent to this discussion is that microbial proliferation can be controlled when corticosteroid therapy is combined with antimicrobial therapy in an individual who has demonstrated adequate immunologic competence. (When an immunologically incompetent individual is under treatment, we recommend preliminary antimicrobial therapy for a sufficient time interval to demonstrate that the therapeutic agent can effectively control the infected microbe. Quantitative bacteriology should prove helpful in such a determination.[25])

In cases where the effectiveness of antimicrobial therapy is questionable (for example, antifungal agents), we have treated the patient first with amphotericin B, nystatin, or pimaricin (experimental drug) simultaneously for about 5 days; then, if the patient is also immunologically competent, we have initiated corticosteroid therapy. (Our experience is limited to two such cases; so we might expect to amend our protocol as we gain more experience.)

In general terms, we have found combined corticosteroid-antimicrobial therapy to be extremely effective in reducing the severity and morbidity of acute corneal stromal infections. We emphasize that each of these studies represents expanded feasibility evaluations. Our controls at best have been sporadic and far removed from the ideal double-blind protocol. Until such studies have transpired, valid effectiveness for this form of therapy cannot be established.

Treatment of peripheral ischemic or corneal disease

Treatment requires reconstitution of the vasculature of the peripheral cornea as well as control of the inflammatory process. The severity of the initial inflammation is adequately severe to interfere with the patency of limbal vasculature, especially the deep limbal complex of vessels. The mechanism by which this reaction occurs most likely begins as a perivasculitis and ends in intravascular clotting. Heparin facilitates reconstitution of vascular patency by preventing new clot formation. Actual clot lysis is most likely effected by the intrinsic fibrinolysins that occur in high concentration in ocular tissues. If one uses corticosteroid therapy in conjunction with heparin, the severe inflammatory response that sets up the initial vascular reaction can be controlled. In our experience this combination of therapeutic agents has produced excellent results.

Recurrent inflammation in corticosteroid-treated cases

Inflammatory recurrence has been evaluated only in infiltrative corneal disease patients. It should be stressed that inflammatory recurrence does not necessarily mean that the initial infectious agent, that is, herpes simplex virus, is responsible for the recurrent episode. For example, herpes simplex stromal keratitis represented 67% of all patients followed for the 1-year posttreatment period; 63% of these patients demonstrated a recurrent inflammatory episode but only three patients (9%) demonstrated a dendrite. Virus cultures were not performed; so atypical herpesvirus involvement cannot be ruled out. It is especially important to note that these herpes recurrence figures should not be directly compared with recurrence rates of epithelial herpes infection reported by Carroll and others[26] and by Jones.[27] The patients in those series showed no evidence of stromal disease, and recurrence was diagnosed on the reappearance of the epithelial dendrite or other significant clinical signs. However, the rate of recurrent inflammation in corticosteroid-treated corneal stromal disease is exceptionally high. Whether corticosteroid therapy plays a role in predisposing to recurrent inflammation cannot be evaluated at this time.

We have been particularly interested in the role of structural alteration in predisposing to subsequent inflammation. Experimentally, a severe corneal lesion enhances vascular permeability markedly in contrast to a mild lesion.[28] Such change in corneal vascular permeability predisposes to recurrent inflammation by establishing an acquired host hyperreactivity to exogenous stimuli.[29] Our clinical series have clearly demonstrated that patients with severely altered corneas show a much greater incidence of recurrence than do patients with mild structural change.

A similar phenomenon occurs in peripheral corneal infiltrative disease. Patients with peripheral vascular changes (pannus) invariably demonstrate recurrent inflammation, while patients who remain free of secondary neovascularization remain stable. The ocular literature contains numerous references to such phenomena in descriptions of the relentless progression of vernal, rosacea, and trachomatous keratoconjunctivitis.

The penetrating keratoplasty seems to play a significant role in reducing the predilection of altered corneal structure to recurrent inflammation. Structurally, the graft provides a clear postsurgical cornea that replaces neovascularized scar tissue. Regardless of diagnosis, the overall incidence of recurrent inflammation has been reduced almost three times. Another study of the keratoplasty has disclosed that delayed graft reactions (inflammatory recurrence) invariably occur in patients with heavily vascularized host cornea beds, again without regard to cause. This finding has prompted us to examine patients in this structural category at much more frequent intervals than patients with minimally vascularized host corneas.

Obviously, we cannot discount experimental and clinical data that clearly demonstrate the predilection of the infected patient to incur repeated infections with the initially presenting microbe. These data are particularly tenable in herpes simplex virus[30-32] and *Staphylococcus.*[33] It seems likely that the synergistic reaction of a given microbe and structural alteration leads to inflammatory recurrence. *Both* factors must be controlled if optimal long-term results are to be achieved.

Finally, we must consider the startling difference in long-term success rates between indigent (S.F.G.H.) and private patients. We have attempted to isolate the factors that predispose our indigent patients to recurrent inflammation. The only factor common to every indigent individual was isolation from his environment during active therapy (hospitalization). Control of this situation is beyond the scope of a corneal treatment group; we frankly do not know how to cope with this situation. Whether this factor is significant in other long-term corneal series cannot be evaluated at this time.

SUMMARY

This study presents the results of combined high-dosage topical corticosteroid-antimicrobial therapy in infiltrative corneal disease, which we have divided into central stromal keratitis and peripheral corneal infiltrative disease. Of the 146 stromal keratitis patients treated on the combined regimen, 98% demonstrated improvement; 44% achieved a VA of greater than 20/40. Seventy-four patients in this group went on to require a penetrating keratoplasty; of these, 70% achieved a successful graft, 60% with a VA of greater than 20/40. In the acute peripheral infiltrative group, 32 patients (50 eyes), or 92%, demonstrated improvement on combined therapy.

Also included in this study are the results of combined corticosteroid-heparin therapy in syndromes that we have designated as infectious peripheral ischemic disease. Of the nine eyes (eight patients) treated on this regimen, all nine, or 100%, demonstrated marked improvement.

REFERENCES

1. Gordon, D. M.: Prednisone and prednisolone in ocular disease, Amer. J. Ophthal. **41**:593, 1956.
2. Kaufman, H. E., and Maloney, E. D.: IDU and hydrocortisone in experimental herpes simplex keratitis, Arch. Ophthal. **68**:396, 1962.
3. Thygeson, P.: IUDR and simplex keratitis in San Francisco. In Kimura, S. J., and Goodner, E. K., editors: Ocular pharmacology and therapeutics and the problems of medical management, Philadelphia, 1963, F. A. Davis Co., pp. 222-231.
4. Jawetz, E., and others: Studies on herpes simplex. X: The effect of corticosteroids on herpetic keratitis in the rabbit, J. Immun. **83**:486, 1959.
5. Aronson, S. B., and Moore, T. E., Jr.: Corticosteroid therapy in central stromal keratitis, Amer. J. Ophthal. **67**:873, 1969.
6. Aronson, S. B., Elliott, J. H., and others: Pathogenetic approach to therapy of peripheral corneal inflammatory disease, Amer. J. Ophthal. **70**:65, 1970.
7. Ward, P. A., Cochrane, C. G., and Muller-Eberhard, J. H.: The role of serum complement in chemotaxis of leukocytes in vitro, J. Exp. Med. **122**:327, 1965.
8. Aronson, S. B., Sussman, S. J., and others: Corticosteroid therapy in metastatic endophthalmitis, Arch. Ophthal. **85**:61, 1971.
9. Aronson, S. B., and Moore, T. E., Jr.: Serum immunoglobulin testing in corneal disease, Arch. Ophthal. (In preparation.)
10. Hirsch, J. G., and Cohn, Z. A.: Degranulation of polymorphonuclear leukocytes following phagocytosis of microorganisms, J. Exp. Med. **112**:1005, 1960.
11. Thomas, L.: Possible role of leukocyte granules in the Schwartzman and Arthus reaction, Proc. Soc. Exp. Biol. Med. **115**:235, 1964.
12. Swan, K. C., and others: Subepithelial versus subcapsular injection of drugs, Arch. Ophthal. **56**:26, 1956.
13. Hynduik, R. A., and Reagan, M. G.: Radioactive depot-corticosteroid penetration into monkey ocular tissue, Arch. Ophthal. **80**:499, 1968.
14. Levine, N. D., and Aronson, S. B.: Orbital infusion of steroids in the rabbit, Arch. Ophthal. **83**:599, 1970.
15. Bloome, M. A., and others: Antibiotic concentration in ocular tissue, Arch. Ophthal. **83**:78, 1969.
16. Jawetz, E., and others: Studies on herpes simplex, J. Immun. **95**:635, 1965.
17. Laibson, P. R., and Kilbrick, S.: Reactivation of herpetic keratitis in the rabbit. II. Repeated reactivation in the same host, Arch. Ophthal. **77**:254, 1967.
18. Dawson, C. R., and others: Structural changes in chronic herpetic keratitis, Arch. Ophthal. **79**:740, 1968.
19. Harbin, T.: Recurrence of a corneal Pseudomonas infection: after topical steroid therapy, Amer. J. Ophthal. **58**:670, 1964.
20. Michael, M., Jr., and others: Course of experimental tuberculosis in the albino rat as influenced by cortisone, Proc. Soc. Exp. Biol. Med. **75**:613, 1950.
21. Editorial: Cortisone and ACTH in tuberculosis, Lancet **2**:632, 1950.
22. Thomas, L., and Mogabgab, W. J.: Hemorrhagic skin lesions produced by intradermal Meningococcus toxin in rabbits following treatment with ACTH or cortisone, Proc. Soc. Exp. Biol. Med. **74**:829, 1950.
23. Mitsui, Y., and Hamabusa, J.: Corneal infections after cortisone therapy, Brit. J. Ophthal. **39**:244, 1955.
24. Long, D. A.: The influence of corticosteroids on immunological responses to bacterial infection, Int. Arch. Allerg. **105**:5, 1957.
25. Hadley, W. K., and Aronson, S. B.: Quantitative bacteriology of the conjunctiva. Presented at the Association for Research in Ophthalmology, Pacific Section Meeting, Tahoe City, California, September 6, 1969.
26. Carroll, J. M., and others: The recurrence of herpetic keratitis following idoxuridine therapy, Amer. J. Ophthal. **63**:103, 1967.

27. Jones, B. R.: Prospects in treating viral disease of the eye, Trans. Ophthal. Soc. U.K. **87**:537, 1967.
28. Aronson, S. B., Fish, M. B., and others: Altered ocular vascular permeability following inflammation, Arch. Ophthal. **85**:455, 1971.
29. Moore, T. E., Jr., and Aronson, S. B.: The corneal graft: a multi-variable analysis of the penetrating keratoplasty (a monograph), Amer. J. Ophthal. **72**:201, 1971.
30. Kaufman, H. E., and others: Herpes virus in the lacrimal gland, conjunctiva, and cornea of man—a chronic infection, Amer. J. Ophthal. **65**:32, 1968.
31. Nesburn, A. B., and others: Spontaneous reactivation of experimental herpes simplex keratitis in rabbits, Arch. Ophthal. **75**:523, 1967.
32. Laibson, P. R., and Kilbrick, S.: Reactivation of herpetic keratitis by epinephrine in the rabbit, Arch. Ophthal. **75**:254, 1966.
33. Bettman, J. W., Jr., and Aronson, S. B.: Host response in infectious ocular disease: a correlative study between disease severity and circulating immunoglobulins in blepharoconjunctivitis, Arch. Ophthal. **82**:30, 1969.

Chapter 10

Intraocular pressure effects of diluted and new topical corticosteroids

Steven M. Podos, M.D., and Bernard Becker, M.D.

Topically administered corticosteroids produce ocular hypertension in certain susceptible individuals.[1, 2] Three populations, based upon different levels of intraocular pressure response, are described in this chapter. The degree of response to topical corticosteroids is genetically determined. Certain findings that increase the probability of high response of intraocular pressure to topical corticosteroids include the presence of primary open-angle glaucoma, a family history of primary open-angle glaucoma, myopia of high degree, Krukenberg's spindle, and diabetes mellitus.

The variability of the production of corticosteroid-induced ocular hypertension relates not only to the individual but also to the specific compound, its concentration, route of administration, and frequency and duration of application. Dexamethasone 0.1% appears to be more effective in raising intraocular pressure than prednisone 0.12%.[3] Other newer agents, such as medrysone 1.0% and tetrahydrotriamcinolone 0.25%, rarely elevate intraocular pressure. One study describes 11 patients with a mean elevation of 11.8 mm. Hg after 6 weeks of topical betamethasone 0.1% administration, and virtually no rise following treatment with medrysone 1.0%; tetrahydrotriamcinolone 0.25% is similarly without effect in eight subjects whose mean elevation after betamethasone 0.1% is 14.7 mm. Hg.[4]

This study was supported in part by research grant EY 00336 from the National Eye Institute, National Institutes of Health, Bethesda, Maryland.

Table 10-1. Elevation of applanation intraocular pressure after various dilutions of topical dexamethasone*

	Number of patients		
Dexamethasone	*< 6 mm. Hg*	*6 to 15 mm. Hg*	*> 15 mm. Hg*
0.1%	—	—	7
0.05%	—	6	1
0.01%	7	—	—

Adapted from Armaly, M. F.: Steroids and glaucoma. In symposium on glaucoma: transactions of the New Orleans Academy of Ophthalmology, St. Louis, 1967, The C. V. Mosby Co.
*All agents applied three times a day for 4 weeks.

The concentration of the drug plays a role in the magnitude of response. The effect of different concentrations of dexamethasone on the same seven subjects is first compared in Armaly's[2] study, in which a dose-response relationship is demonstrated. The results indicate that the intraocular pressure does not rise more than 5 mm. Hg after 4 weeks of dexamethasone 0.01% (a ten-times dilution of the standard preparation) given three times a day to subjects who are highly sensitive to the 0.1% dexamethasone (Table 10-1). A two-times dilution, 0.05%, gives intermediate findings.

We have compared the responses of 24 patients, all of whom developed intraocular pressures greater than 31 mm. Hg on topical administration of dexamethasone 0.1%, to dexamethasone 0.005% (a twenty-times dilution) and medrysone 1.0%. A similar course of dexamethasone 0.001% (a one-hundred times dilution of the standard preparation) was given to those who had greater than a 5 mm. Hg rise of intraocular pressure when receiving dexamethasone 0.005%. For each individual, the duration of administration was the same for all agents, but the durations varied from one subject to the next from 2 to 6 weeks (mean 4.2 weeks), as determined by the time interval required for the intraocular pressure to exceed 31 mm. Hg while the patient was receiving dexamethasone 0.1%. Frequency of application was four times a day for all patients and all agents. Adequate periods of rest were given between testings to ensure return of intraocular pressure to baseline values. The number of patients who had applanation intraocular pressure elevations either less than 6 mm. Hg, 6 to 15 mm. Hg, or greater than 15 mm. Hg were tabulated for each agent (Table 10-2). The dexamethasone 0.005% produced a rise of intraocular pressure greater than 5 mm. Hg in 11 and greater than 15 mm. Hg in 2 of the 24 patients. The dexamethasone 0.001% or medrysone 1.0% resulted in moderate elevations in only two patients, each of whom responded to dexamethasone 0.005% with at least a 10 mm. Hg rise. One person had a 6 to 15 mm. Hg response to medrysone but not to

Table 10-2. Elevation of applanation intraocular pressure after various dilutions of topical corticosteroids in 24 patients with > 31 mm. Hg after dexamethasone 0.1%*

	Number of patients		
Drug	*< 6 mm. Hg*	*6 to 15 mm. Hg*	*> 15 mm. Hg*
Dexamethasone			
0.1%	—	2	22
0.005%	13	9	2
0.001%	22	2	—
Medrysone			
1.0%	22	2	—

*Duration of therapy for each patient was the same for all agents, four times a day for 2 to 6 weeks (mean 4.2 weeks).

Table 10-3. Applanation intraocular pressure of 24 patients after various topical corticosteroids*

	Number of patients > 31 mm. Hg
No drug	1
Dexamethasone	
0.1%	24
0.005%	10
0.001%	5
Medrysone	
1.0%	4

*Duration of therapy for each patient was the same for all agents, four times a day for 2 to 6 weeks (mean 4.2 weeks).

Table 10-4. Mean applanation intraocular pressure of 24 patients after various corticosteroids*

	Mean intraocular pressure (mm. Hg)
No drug	22.8
Dexamethasone	
0.1%	43.4
0.005%	29.8
Medrysone	
1.0%	24.2

*Duration of topical therapy for each patient was the same for all agents, intraocular pressure > 31 mm. Hg after dexamethasone 0.1% four times a day for 2 to 6 weeks.

dexamethasone 0.001%, and another responded in the opposite manner. An applanation intraocular pressure greater than 31 mm. Hg was present in one patient prior to testing and occurred in ten receiving the 0.005% concentration, five receiving the 0.001% dexamethasone, and four receiving medrysone 1.0% (Table 10-3). The mean intraocular pressures prior to testing and during the various drug treatments for all

Table 10-5. Mean applanation intraocular pressure after various corticosteroids in 11 patients with > 5 mm. Hg rise after dexamethasone 0.005%*

	Mean intraocular pressure (mm. Hg)
No drug	24.0
Dexamethasone	
0.1%	44.7
0.005%	35.9
0.001%	28.6
Medrysone	
1.0%	26.7

*Duration of topical therapy for each patient was the same for all agents, four times a day for 2 to 6 weeks.

24 patients (Table 10-4) and for those 11 responding to dexamethasone 0.005% (Table 10-5) demonstrated a dose-response relationship for the various concentrations of dexamethasone. The least mean elevation was produced by medrysone 1.0%. The mean initial intraocular pressure was similar for those patients with intraocular pressures greater than 31 mm. Hg after treatment with dexamethasone 0.1% and for those more sensitive patients with intraocular pressure elevations greater than 5 mm. Hg after receiving dexamethasone 0.005%.

Duration studies were carried out on some of our subjects. Two of our patients, who had 6 to 15 mm. Hg elevations at the end of 3 weeks of testing, developed greater than 15 mm. Hg rises after 6 weeks of treatment with dexamethasone 0.005%. One patient developed a rise of intraocular pressure in the 6 to 15 mm. Hg range after extended testing with dexamethasone 0.001%. No alteration of response level was produced by maintaining patients receiving medrysone 1.0% up to 6 weeks. No agent was used longer than 6 weeks.

Thus, it appears that a 20-times dilution of dexamethasone 0.1% given topically four times a day for 2 to 6 weeks can provoke significant intraocular pressure elevations in about half of a group of very sensitive patients. If the duration of therapy with diluted dexamethasone is more prolonged, one may expect even greater elevations of intraocular pressure and more intraocular pressure response in patients. Very long-term trials with medrysone 1.0% in patients who are highly sensitive to corticosteroid therapy usually do not produce ocular hypertension (Table 10-6).[5]

Increased frequency of administration also would be expected to alter the results of pharmacologic testing. One study documents an individual receiving betamethasone 0.1% for 8-week periods of once, twice, and four times a day, whose final applanation intraocular pressures are 23, 42, and 55 mm. Hg, respectively.[3] This may account for some

Table 10-6. Use of medrysone for a year in 7 topical corticosteroid responders

	Mean intraocular pressure (mm. Hg)
No steroid	20.2
Steroid	37.7
Medrysone 1.0%	
3 months	20.5
6 months	18.0
12 months	18.1

Adapted from Podos, S. M., Kolker, A. E., and Becker, B.: Topical corticosteroids: dissociation of effects. In Kaufman, H. E., editor: Symposium on ocular anti-inflammatory therapy, Springfield, Ill., 1970, Charles C Thomas, Publisher.

Table 10-7. Case summary of 41-year-old man with blepharoconjunctivitis and corticosteroid-induced glaucoma

	Dosage			
Topical corticosteroid	*Per day*	*Weeks*	*IOP (mm. Hg)*	*Condition*
Hydrocortisone 0.5%	q.i.d.	8	48	Good
None	—	2	21	Bad
Medrysone 1.0%	b.i.d.—q.i.d.	12	18	Better
Dexamethasone 0.001%	q.i.d.	3	16	Worse
Dexamethasone 0.005%	q.i.d.	3	26	Better
Dexamethasone 0.005%	q.i.d.	8	27	

Adapted from Podos, S. M., Kolker, A. E., and Becker, B.: Topical corticosteroids: dissociation of effects. In Kaufman, H. E., editor: Symposium on ocular anti-inflammatory therapy, Springfield, Ill., 1970, Charles C Thomas, Publisher.

of the difference between Armaly's results and those of the present study.

The clinical implications of dose-response studies of corticosteroid-induced intraocular pressure elevations are not completely apparent, because little information exists about the antiinflammatory power of diluted dexamethasone. Dexamethasone 0.005% is found to be effective in a variety of external ocular inflammatory diseases.[6] In one animal model, medrysone 1.0% and dexamethasone 0.001%, but not lesser dilutions, prevented corneal graft reactions.[7] From our data (Table 10-2), these two agents appear to have similar minimal effects on intraocular pressure. Medrysone 1.0% is a weak antiinflammatory drug that is especially useful in the treatment of external ocular disease.[5] With respect to the available compounds, antiinflammatory action generally correlates with intraocular pressure elevation in the susceptible patient. However, in one closely followed patient, medrysone 1.0% but not dexamethasone 0.001% alleviated the symptoms of allergic blepharoconjunctivitis without producing ocular hypertension, while dexamethasone 0.005% elevated intraocular pressure (Table 10-7). Further clinical studies of dexamethasone 0.001% are necessary in order to prove any effect on inflammatory disease similar to the effect produced by the administration of medrysone 1.0%. Corticosteroid drugs that truly dissociate the intraocular pressure and antiinflammatory actions are needed.

REFERENCES

1. Becker, B.: Topical corticosteroids and intraocular pressure. In Becker, B., and Drews, R. C., editors: Current concepts in ophthalmology, vol. 1, St. Louis, 1967, The C. V. Mosby Co.
2. Armaly, M. F.: Steroids and glaucoma. In Symposium on glaucoma, Transactions of the New Orleans Academy of Ophthalmology, St. Louis, 1967, The C. V. Mosby Co.
3. Kayes, J., and Becker, B.: The human trabecular meshwork in corticosteroid-induced glaucoma, Trans. Amer. Ophthal. Soc. **67**:339, 1969.
4. Becker, B., and Kolker, A.: The intraocular pressure response to topical corticosteroids. In Leopold, I. H., editor: Ocular therapy: complications and management, vol. 2, St. Louis, 1967, The C. V. Mosby Co.
5. Podos, S. M., Kolker, A. E., and Becker, B.: Topical corticosteroids: dissociation of effects. In Kaufman, H. E., editor: Symposium on ocular anti-inflammatory therapy, Springfield, Ill., 1970, Charles C Thomas, Publisher.
6. Brown, D. C.: Dexamethasone in human ocular disease and dose-response relationships of some systemic corticosteroids in rabbit xenografts. In Kaufman, H. E., editor: Symposium on ocular anti-inflammatory therapy, Springfield, Ill., 1970, Charles C Thomas, Publisher.
7. Lorenzetti, D. W. C., Ellison, E. M., and Kaufman, H. E.: Quantitative steroid effect on graft reaction, Arch. Ophthal. **79**:64, 1968.

Chapter 11

Individual responsiveness to drugs and pharmacogenetics in ophthalmology

Theodore W. Lieberman, M.D.

The manner in which the individual patient reacts to a drug depends in part on factors that are intrinsic to the individual and that often are genetically determined. The field that encompasses the hereditary patterns of drug responses is known as pharmacogenetics. Although the absorption, distribution, chemical interactions, metabolism, and excretion of all drugs are governed genetically to some extent, the most thoroughly investigated interactions between drug and patient have been instituted in those cases in which unexpected or adverse reactions have occurred. In the field of general pharmacogenetics several such altered reactions have been well studied.[1]

GENERAL PHARMACOGENETICS

Succinylcholine chloride is used as a muscle relaxant in surgery performed under general anesthesia and also in such procedures as electroshock therapy. The drug causes paralysis by depolarization at the neuromuscular junction. It is rapidly metabolized, which limits its duration of action to minutes. Approximately 1 in 3,000 subjects who are administered succinylcholine will have prolonged muscular paralysis and apnea. The pseudocholinesterases of these subjects are often found to hydrolyze succinylcholine to its inactive products at a much slower rate than the pseudocholinesterases found in normal re-

This study was supported in part by U. S. Public Health Service research grants EY 00330 and EY 00340 from the National Eye Institute, National Institutes of Health, Bethesda, Maryland.

actors. The slow inactivation of the drug allows it to have a prolonged action at the neuromuscular junction. Family studies of individuals with this defect have shown that the trait is autosomally transmitted. The genetic alteration leads either to pseudocholinesterases with less affinity for succinylcholine and other drugs or to an absence of enzyme activity (silent gene).

Isoniazid, the antituberculosis drug, is mainly inactivated by acetylation, a reaction catalyzed by the liver enzyme acetyl transferase. Lack of this enzyme leads to increased body concentrations of isoniazid and an increased incidence of toxic side effects, especially peripheral neuropathies. Slow inactivation of isoniazid is an autosomally transmitted recessive trait requiring the patient who clinically manifests this defect to be homozygous with respect to the genes governing slow inactivation. Patients who are heterozygotes have sufficient acetyl transferase to metabolize isoniazid at a fast enough rate to prevent toxicities at the usual therapeutic dosage level of isoniazid.

Other examples of genetically related drug responses in general pharmacology include hemolytic anemias induced by drugs administered to patients with sex-linked glucose-6-phosphate dehydrogenase deficiencies; a dominant, autosomally transmitted resistance to coumarin anticoagulation; and the induction of acute attacks of porphyria by the administration of barbiturates to susceptible patients.

PHARMACOGENETICS IN OPHTHALMOLOGY

Corticosteroid responsiveness

In ophthalmology several examples of pharmacogenetics also exist. The most thoroughly investigated and well-known of these reactions is the elevation of intraocular pressure that occurs in susceptible individuals after the prolonged topical administration of potent corticosteroids. Table 11-1, from the work of Becker and associates,[2] demonstrates the familial nature of this response. When individuals in the

Table 11-1. Intraocular pressure responses to topical corticosteroid testing

Category	*Applanation pressure* $\geqslant$ *20 mm. Hg*	*Applanation pressure* $>$ *31 mm. Hg*
Volunteers (selected*)	30%	4%
Volunteers (unselected)	38%	6%
Offspring†	90%	22%
Siblings†	78%	26%

Modified from Becker, B.: Topical corticosteroids and intraocular pressure. In Becker, B., and Drews, R. C., editors: Current concepts in ophthalmology, St. Louis, 1967, The C. V. Mosby Co.

*Excluding those with positive water tonograms.

†Offspring and siblings of volunteers with applanation pressures > 31 mm. Hg after corticosteroid provocative test.

general population are administered 0.1% betamethasone or dexamethasone three to four times daily to the eye, approximately 38% of this population will be found to have an intraocular pressure equal to or over 20 mm. Hg, and 4% of the population will have a pressure over 31 mm. Hg after 6 weeks of therapy. The normal intraocular pressure is 15.5 mm. Hg, with a standard deviation of ± 2.5 mm. Hg. As seen in Table 11-1, the siblings and children of subjects from the general population who respond to topical corticosteroid therapy show a higher frequency of response to topical steroids than is found in the general population. Although there is some disagreement as to the exact mode of genetic transmission,[3-6] this evidence strongly supports the concept of hereditability of this characteristic. The trait is considered by most authorities to be autosomally transmitted. Heterozygotes have less of a pressure response to topical steroids than individuals homozygous for the trait have. A very high incidence of steroid responsiveness as compared with a volunteer population has been demonstrated in subjects with chronic simple glaucoma,[7] in their relatives, and in individuals with Krukenberg's spindles,[8] nonproliferative diabetic retinopathy,[9] and myopia of over five diopters.[10] Special precautions should be taken to monitor the intraocular pressure during the use of topical corticosteroids in patients fitting in the above categories.

Drug sensitivity in Down's syndrome

Children with Down's syndrome have been found to have an increased sensitivity to the mydriatic effect of locally applied atropine.[11-13] Fig. 11-1 is a graph of the average pupillary diameter increase with time after the instillation of 1% atropine sulfate into the conjunctival sac. In this experiment[12] 30 subjects with Down's syndrome were matched with regard to age, sex, intelligence, and iris color to 30 subjects without Down's syndrome. The difference between the pupillary responses of the two groups to atropine was significant. It was suggested that this hypersensitivity resulted from a hypoplasia of the iris stroma. Lowe[14] has found 95% of 67 individuals with Down's syndrome to have this iris characteristic.

In 1957 Walsh[15] and McKusick[16] both commented on the sensitivity of children with Down's syndrome to atropine, mentioning that fatalities from its use have been reported. In 1967, Harris and Goodman[17] showed an increased sensitivity in individuals with Down's syndrome to the cardioaccelerator effect of atropine (Fig. 11-2). This suggests that the previously observed increased iris sensitivity was caused by more than a local anatomical alteration. The explanation of this sensitivity appears to be more complex than just a supersensitivity of the receptor site to atropine or decreased destruction of atropine. Atropine increases

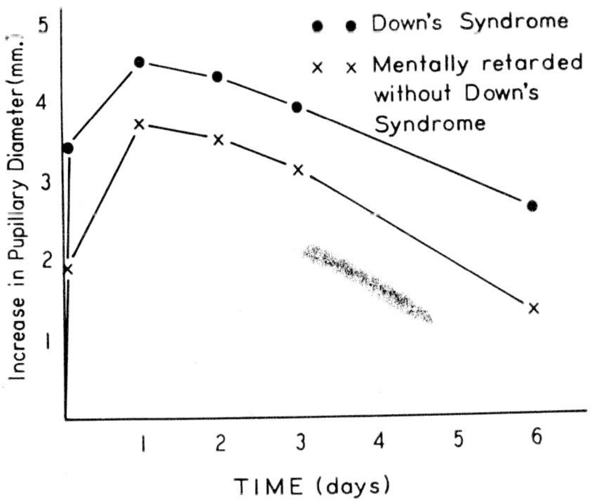

Fig. 11-1. Average increase in pupillary diameter with time after instillation of 1% atropine sulfate into conjunctival cul-de-sac (see text for details). (Modified from Priest, J. H.: J. Dis. Child. **100**:869, 1960.)

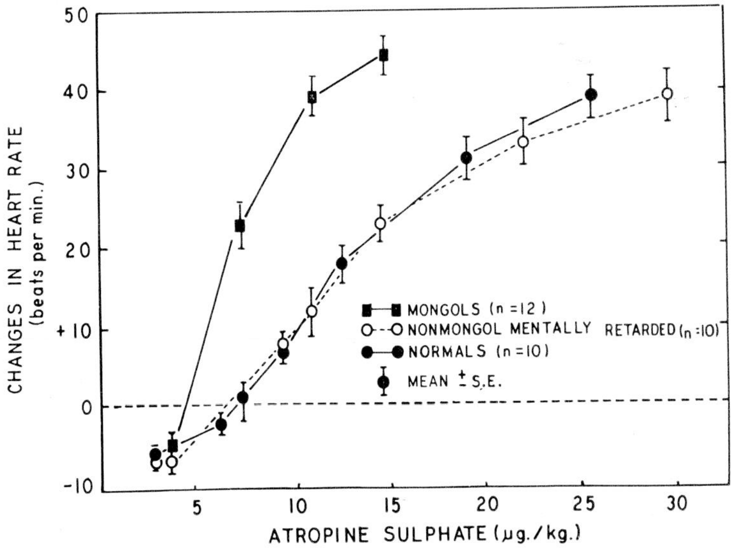

Fig. 11-2. Increase in heart rate after increasing increments of intravenous atropine sulfate. (From Harris, W. S., and Goodman, R. M.: New Eng. J. Med. **279**:407, 1968.)

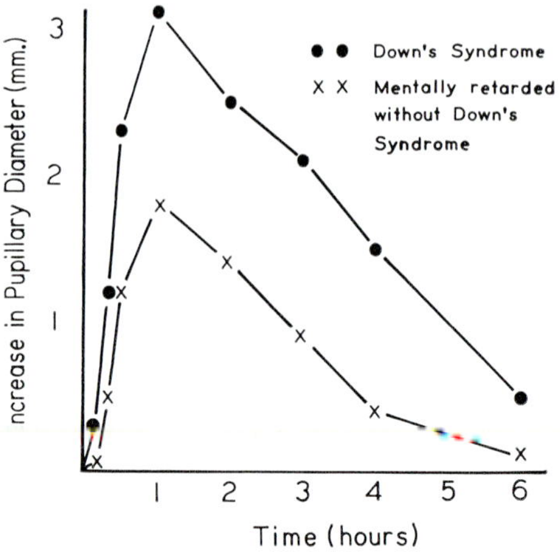

Fig. 11-3. Average increase in pupillary diameter with time in 30 individuals with Down's syndrome and in 30 mentally retarded individuals without Down's syndrome after instillation of 1% hydroxyamphetamine hydrobromide into the conjunctival cul-de-sac. (Modified from Priest, J. H.: J. Dis. Child. **100**:869, 1960.)

the heart rate by blocking the parasympathetic slowing effect of the vagus nerve. However, in Down's syndrome, propranolol hydrochloride, a β-sympathetic blocker, abolishes most of the cardioaccelerator sensitivity to atropine.[17] Individuals with this chromosomal abnormality have also been reported to be supersensitive to the mydriatic effects of hydroxyamphetamine (Paredrine[12]) hydrobromide (Fig. 11-3). Elsewhere in this symposium Apt (Chapter 2) has reported a supersensitivity of children with Down's syndrome to anticholinesterases.

Racial or pigmentary influence on drug responsiveness

In 1927 Howard and Lee[18] noted that individuals with darker irides reacted with less of a mydriatic response to ephedrine than patients with light irides. This study was performed in China; and the individuals with light irides were all Caucasians while those with darker irides were Chinese. Independently in 1927, while working with ephedrine, Chen noted that when he instilled the agent into his own eyes, the response was much less brisk than he had found using the drug in an experiment on a Caucasian population. Chen and Poth[19] studied the effect of a number of topical agents on mydriasis and found the irides of Negroes to be least responsive to these agents, the irides of Chinese to be intermediate in response, and the irides of Caucasians to be most responsive (Table 11-2). Fig. 11-4 shows the difference in response to cocaine of a blue-eyed Caucasian female and a heavily pigmented Negro female. It is interesting that

Table 11-2. Average increase in pupillary diameter (mm.) after topical mydriatic administration, according to race

	Race		
Drug	Caucasians (10*)	Chinese (10*)	Negroes (10*)
l-ephedrine	2.2	0.6	0.3
d,l-ephedrine	1.7	0.3	0.2
d-pseudoephedrine	0.8	0.2	0.1
cocaine	2.0	0.7	0.3
eucatropine	2.2	0.7	0.2

Adapted from Chen, K. K., and Poth, E. J.: Racial differences as illustrated by the mydriatic action of cocaine, euphthalmine, and ephedrine, J. Pharm. Exp. Ther. **36**:429, 1929.
*Number of subjects.

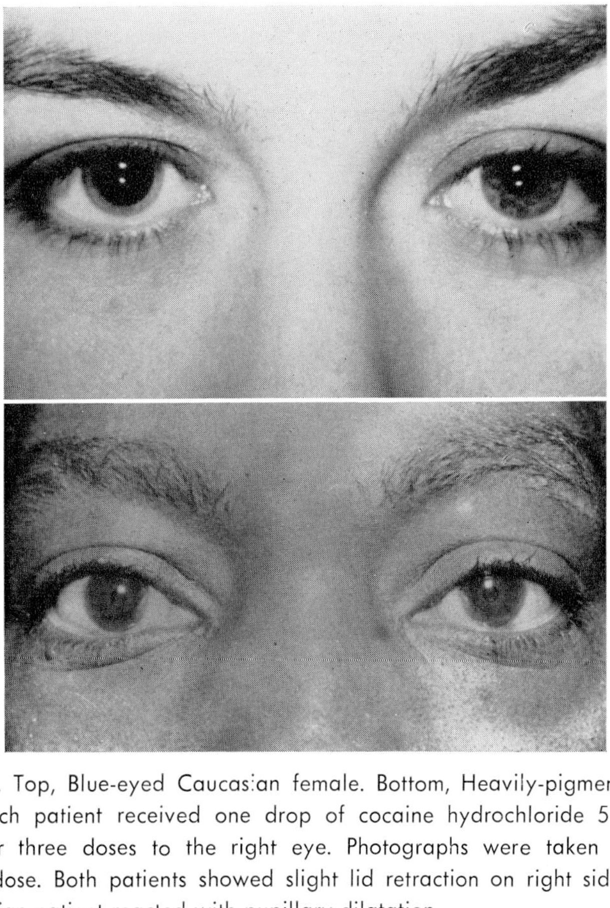

Fig. 11-4. Top, Blue-eyed Caucasian female. Bottom, Heavily-pigmented Negro female. Each patient received one drop of cocaine hydrochloride 5% every 5 minutes for three doses to the right eye. Photographs were taken 45 minutes after last dose. Both patients showed slight lid retraction on right side, but only the Caucasian patient reacted with pupillary dilatation.

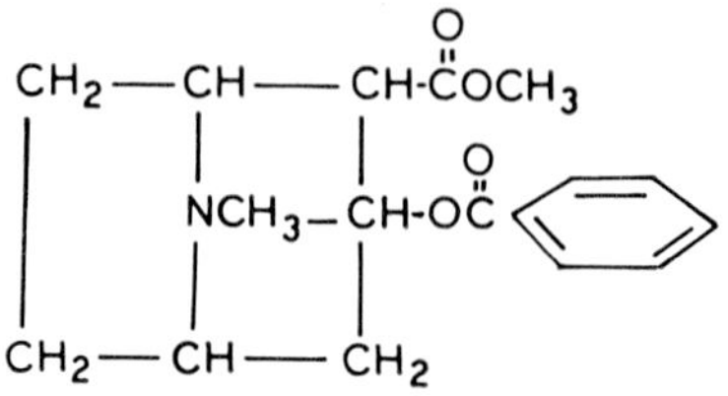

COCAINE

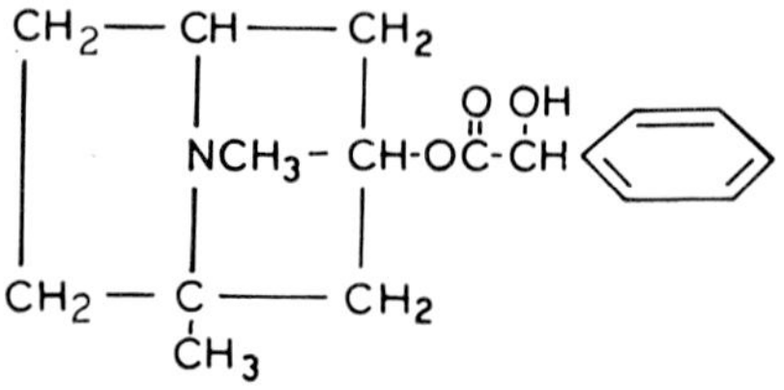

EUCATROPINE

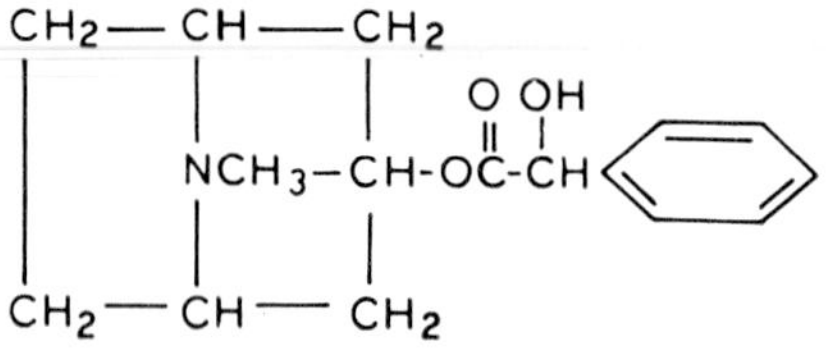

HOMATROPINE

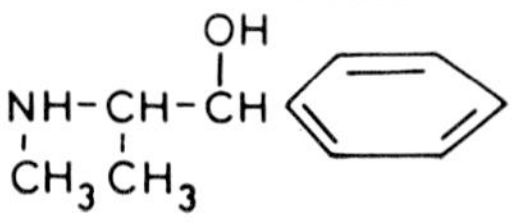

EPHEDRINE

Fig. 11-5. Molecular formulas of various compounds that on local administration to the eye show less mydriatic effect in Negroes than in Caucasians.

the cocaine test for Horner's syndrome depends on the pupillary dilatation in the eye with an intact sympathetic system. It is obvious that the test is of no value in heavily pigmented Negroes. Eucatropine hydrochloride, which has been suggested as a good drug for performing mydriatic provocative tests in subjects with anatomical narrow angles, will show little reactivity in the Negro. Scott[20] found a similar lack of response to homatropine hydrobromide in the eye of the West African Negro. We believe that a decreased mydriatic response to epinephrine is present in darkly pigmented individuals.

Chen and Poth[19] explained the lack of responsiveness of the heavily pigmented iris on the basis of a mechanical interference with dilatation caused by the large number of pigment granules in the iris melanocytes. We are presently investigating other mechanisms that might be responsible for this difference in response. The structural formulas for many of these compounds except for the ephedrine and epinephrine groups are similar (Fig. 11-5). It has been known for many years that certain rabbits have an enzyme that breaks down atropine (atropine esterase).[21] More recently a cocaine esterase has been described,[22] and these two enzymes have been shown to differ from each other.[23] Mr. J. Nowakowski and I have examined the sera of patients whose irides were both responsive and unresponsive to cocaine for the presence of esterases in the unresponsive patients. In thin layer chromato-

Table 11-3. Difference in pressure and outflow facility between treated and untreated eyes in normal Caucasians and Negroes two hours after treatment with 4% pilocarpine and 2% epinephrine

	Number of eyes	*T appl. mm. Hg*	P_o *mm. Hg*	*C µl/min/mm. Hg*
4% pilocarpine				
Caucasians	15	−1.1	−1.8	+0.10
Negroes	11	−0.4	−0.9	+0.05
2% epinephrine				
Caucasians	15	−1.3	0.0	+0.12
Negroes	11	−0.3	+1.1	+0.05

graphic techniques, incubations of the sera with cocaine for 24 hours at 37° C. have shown no differences in the breakdown of cocaine in either group.

Another possible mechanism for lack of responsiveness that is presently under investigation is that the pigment granules absorb the drug and compete with the pharmacologic receptors for the agent. Potts[24] has shown that many drugs, especially the polycyclic compounds, are strongly absorbed by pigment granules.

A more important problem relates to glaucoma control. In drug-testing experiments using epinephrine as a comparison drug, we have noted that the more heavily pigmented volunteers did not always react as well as lightly pigmented individuals to the antiglaucoma (intraocular pressure and outflow facility) effects. Dr. Melikian, Dr. Leopold, and I[25] have tested this observation more critically by investigating the effects of 2% epinephrine (and in other experiments 4% pilocarpine hydrochloride) on the intraocular pressure and outflow facilities in a group of healthy female volunteers who were free of eye disease. The subjects were graded as to skin, iris, trabeculum, and fundus pigmentation. The response to these drugs was evaluated 2 hours after instillation. The heavily pigmented individuals were found to be less responsive than the lightly pigmented group. Most of the heavily pigmented subjects were Negroes; therefore, it cannot be determined from this experiment whether the differences were racially determined independent of pigmentation or solely on the amount of pigment present in the eye. Table 11-3 shows the difference between the reaction of Negroes and Caucasians to these two drugs on an acute experimental basis.

A deeper understanding of the genetic responses to drugs is important in all fields of medicine. It not only helps the clinician in his choice of therapy but also in his understanding of the individual response. New therapies that are specifically related to these pharmacogenetic problems are already being developed.

REFERENCES

1. Goldstein, A., Aronow, L., and Kalman, S. M.: Principle of drug action, the basis of pharmacology, New York, Harper & Row, Publishers, 1969, pp. 271-273, 429-475.
2. Becker, B.: Topical corticosteroids and intraocular pressure. In Becker, B., and Drews, R. C., editors: Current concepts in ophthalmology, St. Louis, 1967, The C. V. Mosby Co., pp. 132-147.
3. Armaly, M. F., Monstavicius, B. F., and Sayegh, R. E.: Ocular pressure and aqueous outflow facility in siblings, Arch. Ophthal. **80**:354, 1968.
4. Francois, J., Heintz-de Bree, C. H., and Tripathi, R. C.: The cortisone test and the heredity of primary open-angle glaucoma, Amer. J. Ophthal. **62**:844, 1966.
5. Spaeth, G. L.: Effects of topical dexamethasone on intraocular pressure and the water drinking test, Arch. Ophthal. **76**:778, 1966.
6. Levene, R., Wigdor, A., and others: Topical corticosteroids in normal patients and glaucoma suspects, Arch. Ophthal. **77**:593, 1967.
7. Becker, B., and Mills, D. W.: Elevated intraocular pressure following corticosteroid eye drops, J.A.M.A. **185**:884, 1963.
8. Becker, B., and Podos, S. M.: Krukenberg's spindles and primary open-angle glaucoma, Arch. Ophthal. **76**:635, 1966.
9. Becker, B., Bresnick, G., and others: The intraocular pressure and its response to topical corticosteroids in diabetes, Arch. Ophthal. **76**:477, 1966.
10. Podos, S. M., Becker, B., and Morton, W. R.: High myopia and primary open-angle glaucoma, Amer. J. Ophthal. **62**:1039, 1966.
11. Berg, J. M., Brandon, M. W. G., and Kirman, B. H.: Atropine in mongolism, Lancet **2**:441, 1959.
12. Priest, J. H.: Atropine response of eyes in mongolism, Amer. J. Dis. Child **100**:869, 1960.
13. O'Brien, D., Haake, M. W., and Braid, B.: Atropine sensitivity and serotonin in mongolism, Amer. J. Dis. Child **100**:873, 1960.
14. Lowe, R. F.: Eye in mongolism, Brit. J. Ophthal. **33**:131, 1949.
15. Walsh, F. B.: Clinical neuro-ophthalmology, ed. 2, Baltimore, 1957, The Williams and Wilkins Co., p. 1192.
16. McKusick, V. A.: Symposium on inborn errors of metabolism: mechanisms in genetic diseases of man, Amer. J. Med. **22**:676, 1957.
17. Harris, W. S., and Goodman, R. M.: Hyper-reactivity to atropine in Down's syndrome, New Eng. J. Med. **279**:407, 1968.
18. Howard, H. J., and Lee, T. P.: The effect of instillations of ephedrine solution upon the eye, Proc. Soc. Exp. Biol. Med. **24**:700, 1927.
19. Chen, K. K., and Poth, E. J.: Racial differences as illustrated by the mydriatic action of cocaine, euphthalmine, and ephedrine, J. Pharmacol. Exp. Ther. **36**:429, 1929.
20. Scott, J. G.: The eye of the West African Negro, Brit. J. Ophthal. **29**:12, 1945.
21. Sawin, P. B., and Glick, D.: Atropinesterase, a genetically determined enzyme in the rabbit, Proc. Nat. Acad. Sci. U.S.A. **29**:55, 1943.
22. Werner, G.: Fermentdefekte als ursache unterschiedlicher mydriatischer wirksamkeit von atropin und cocain bei kaninchen, Naunyn-Schmiedeberg Arch. Pharm. Exp. Path. **251**:320, 1965.
23. Stormont, C., and Suzuki, Y.: Atropinesterase and cocainesterase of rabbit serum: localization of the enzyme activity in isozymes, Science **167**:200, 1970.
24. Potts, A. M.: The reaction of uveal pigment in vitro with polycyclic compounds, Invest. Ophthal. **3**:405, 1964.
25. Melikian, H. E., Lieberman, T. W., and Leopold, I. H.: Ocular pigmentation and pressure and outflow responses to pilocarpine and epinephrine, Amer. J. Ophthal. **72**:70, 1971.

Chapter 12

Effectiveness study of antibiotics

Robert P. Burns, M.D.

Controversy over the effectiveness of antibiotic prophylaxis against postoperative infection has existed since the antibiotic era began 25 years ago. Consensus, which has tended to favor the use of preoperative antibiotics, is supported by analysis of results of a large series of cataract operations.[1, 2] There is less agreement relating to the best mode or time of delivery of antibiotics or the most effective antibiotic. Many opinions have been voiced, but factual data are lacking. For this reason this study was begun.

It has been known since the time of Axenfeld[3] that bandaging the eye raises the local temperature and increases bacterial growth. After cataract surgery, the incubator effect of the bandage, the devascularization of the conjunctival flap, the implantation of sutural foreign bodies, the immobilization of the cleansing action of the eyelids and lacrimal pump by the bandage, and the possible obstruction of the lacrimal canaliculi by ointment medication all contribute to an increase in bacterial count in the human eye.[4]

Utilizing these observations, a quantitative technique to determine bacterial multiplication from the preoperative to postoperative phase was devised in order that different types of antibiotics or treatment

This study was supported in part by research grant 5 RO1-A102763-11 from the National Institute of Allergy and Infectious Diseases, Department of Health, Education, and Welfare, Washington, D. C.

I am deeply indebted to members of the resident staff of the University of Oregon Medical School, Department of Ophthalmology for their enthusiastic cooperation in this study of their patients. Mrs. Marilyn Oden did the bacterial counts, and Dr. Virginia Weimar and Miss Jean Troudt did the statistical analyses.

methods could be evaluated.[4] Preoperative and postoperative bacterial counts were done by rubbing a cotton swab over a standardized area of the lower palpebral conjunctiva, the lower lid margin, and the inner canthus. The swab was immersed for a few minutes in a 0.1% solution of a nonionic surfactant detergent (Triton X-100) in nutrient broth and was shaken to break up the bacterial clumps by detergent action. An aliquot of the detergent-broth mixture was diluted serially by pipetting 0.1 ml. of detergent blood mixture into 0.9 ml. of sterile nutrient broth in several successive tubes, and the bacteria were then counted by conventional dilution pour plate techniques. The plate containing 30 to 300 colonies of bacteria was the one recorded, with the result multiplied by the dilution factor to obtain the total number of bacteria in the eye sample. Complicated cases of cataract surgery were excluded. Such quantitative bacterial counts have been used frequently in the study of other diseased areas where some bacteria might normally be expected, such as in the urinary or pulmonary tracts.

The first evaluation done was a double-blind study of antibiotic ointments applied to the eye both at the time of surgery and after surgery.[4] Gentamicin sulfate 0.3% ointment was compared both with neomycin sulfate 0.5% ointment and with a "lubricating ointment" utilized as a placebo.[4] Of 21 gentamicin-treated eyes, 3 showed a postoperative increase in bacterial count and 18 showed a decrease. Of 27 neomycin-treated eyes, 2 showed no change from preoperative to postoperative count, 12 showed an increase in bacterial count, and 13 showed a decrease. With the nonmedicated lubricant (control) ointment 16 of 18 eyes showed an increase in bacterial count postoperatively, and only 2 showed a decrease. These data were clear. Both neomycin and gentamicin were statistically more effective than the unmedicated lubricant, but gentamicin was more effective than neomycin.

In a continuation of this study we have evaluated the effect of variation in frequency, type, and delivery of antibiotic medication. The double-blind technique and placebo controls were not considered necessary, since the discrepancy between treated and nontreated eyes is so great.[4] The first bacteria count was done 1 or 2 days preoperatively and repeated 2 or 3 days postoperatively. A consecutive series of patients was studied with each drug until a significant number was attained.

The first antibiotic tested was gentamicin. Twenty mg. (volume, 0.5 ml.) were given subconjunctivally at 6 o'clock at the end of cataract surgery. The second antibiotic tested was chloramphenicol ophthalmic ointment 1% applied only once to the lower conjunctival cul-de-sac at the end of the operation. The third antibiotic tested was gentamicin ophthalmic ointment 0.3%. It was applied four times daily for 1 or

Table 12-1. Effectiveness study of antibiotics

	Subconjunctival gentamicin		*Chloramphenicol ointment*		*Gentamicin ointment*	
	Preop.	*Postop.*	*Preop.*	*Postop.*	*Preop.*	*Postop.*
	2,500	20	15,700	410	23,000	0
	2,600	60	1,170	1,310	1,200	0
	310	0	1,500	1,160	700	0
	280	7	260	170	3,600	0
	1,900	20	30,000	320	14,900	0
	350	3,000	1,150	19,500	2,100	0
	11	2	730	3,700	33,700	0
	51	0	5,600	1,830	1,200	0
	4,000	1	2,250	0	1,600	0
	150	70	1,100	5,100	11,100	2,060
	13,000	105	19,500	150	1,000	0
	20	0	14,700	10,500	17,900	0
	4,200	130	1,720	93	100	0
	13	0	8,800	190	900	0
	4,900	140	5,100	11,600	13,500	0
	12,500	3	22,500	67	400	300
	2,100	2	6,400	176	21,000	0
	16,700	10	1,400	181	15,500	0
	210	0	30,000	4,300	3,600	0
	0	0	1,580	140	12,000	0
	4,340	2	340	950	3,400	0
	25	0	50	19	21,000	0
	20,000	2	710	530	15,500	0
	700	10	3,800	11,200	3,600	0
	4,110	3	14,000	4,000	12,000	0
	2,950	8			5,900	1,100
	6,600	217			400	0
	300	3			9,600	0
	300	1,040			3,500	0
	30,000	20			40,000	0
	12,000	30			5,100	0
	650	0			20,000	0
	15,000	10			12,900	0
	430	0			2,500	0
					4,000	0
					32,600	0
Mean	4,800	144	7,842	3,103	10,302	96

2 days preoperatively, placed in the lower conjunctival cul-de-sac at the time of surgery, and put in the eye once daily at the time of dressing change for 2 days (Table 12-1).

To compare drop and ointment dosage forms, the fourth antibiotic tested was a neomycin–polymixin-B–gramicidin drop, which was given with the same frequency as the gentamicin ointment. Next, 30% sulfacetimide, and last, 0.3% gentamicin drop medication were used in similar fashion—4 times daily preoperatively, at the time of surgery, and at daily postoperative dressing changes (Table 12-2).

Table 12-2. Effectiveness study of antibiotics

30% sulfacetimide drops		*Neomycin–polymixin-B–gramicidin drops*		*Gentamicin 0.3% drops*	
Preop.	*Postop.*	*Preop.*	*Postop.*	*Preop.*	*Postop.*
540	20	4,500	204	410	0
22	18,400	140	1,570	130	0
1,150	88	10,000	30,000	20	0
1,950	168	442	0	2,400	30
440	40	7,000	50	300	0
300	520	2,600	6	300	0
2,600	0	3,000	2	1,100	28
108	530	60	0	1,500	0
1,810	146	5,500	0	900	0
20,000	5,300	4,100	0	50,000	0
1,380	15,000	9,200	4	27,600	320
3,500	410	6,100	158	5,800	0
520	22	23,500	10	70,000	0
1,050	1,200	252	20	16,000	28
420	40	76	38	800	0
3,100	1,130	5,700	2	1,710	0
30,000	30,000	11,000	40	160,000	8
206	0	50,000	212	30,000	260
406	32,000	22,000	4,500	31,600	92
800	730	20,000	26	2,800	12
3,900	9,600	18	20	45,000	0
16,100	14,000	2,330	6	1,200	50
10,500	2,660	14,000	26,900	24,000	0
7,800	20,000	22	12	56	16
1,930	2,370	7,300	720	7,400	148
		280	6,000	360	72
		45,700	0	94	6
		80	30,000	870	0
		476	54	100,000	0
		12,800	520	990	0
		2	6	3,400	0
		12,600	0		
		76	30,000		
Mean 4,424	6,175	8,480	3,972	18,936	33

There are great variations in the numbers of bacteria present in the preoperative counts (Tables 12-1 and 12-2). Dr. Virginia Weimar has done a multiple linear regression analysis of these data on a computer and has found that the variability in preoperative figures does not affect the postoperative data. Comparison of results with one drug versus another was done by the analysis of variance technique and by the student T test, although in our previous study[4] comparison of results was done by recording increase or decrease in bacterial count postoperatively (Fig. 12-1). This did not seem to be as valid a tech-

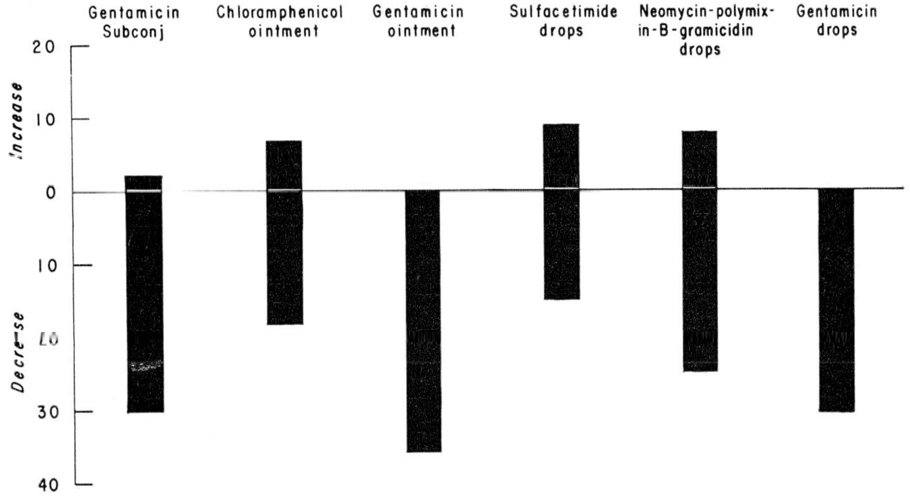

Fig. 12-1. Postoperative bacterial counts compared to preoperative counts.

Table 12-3. Mean bacterial counts

	Administration		*Bacterial count*	
Drug	*Mode*	*Time*	*Preop.*	*Postop.*
Gentamicin 20 mg.	Subconjunctivally	At operation	4,800	144
Chloramphenicol 1%	Ointment	At operation	7,842	3,103
Gentamicin 0.3%	Ointment	4 × daily preop. 1 × daily postop.	10,302	96
Sulfacetimide 30%	Drops	4 × daily preop. 1 × daily postop.	4,424	6,175
Neomycin–polymixin-B–gramicidin	Drops	4 × daily preop. 1 × daily postop.	8,480	3,972
Gentamicin 0.3%	Drops	4 × daily preop. 1 × daily postop.	18,936	33

nique for comparison of the total data as the present methods. Mean counts are listed in Table 12-3.

RESULTS

Gentamicin injected subconjunctivally at the time of surgery was quite effective in keeping the conjunctival sac and lid margin sterile for 2 days. Gentamicin ointment and drops were, however, significantly more effective in reducing the bacterial count than subconjunctival gentamicin. Analysis of variance tests showed that all forms of application of gentamicin were more effective than chloramphenicol 1% ointment applied once at the time of operation. The neomycin–polymixin-B–gramicidin drops and sulfacetimide drops were decreasingly less effective, but these last two groups had so much variance that they were not a valid population for comparison by the analysis of variance test.

There was no statistical difference between the gentamicin ointment or drops by analysis of variance. However, 33 of 36 ointment-treated eyes were free of bacteria on postoperative culture. These are the best results obtained by this criterion, since 12 of 31 gentamicin drop–treated eyes contained bacteria. Bacteria isolated were usually micrococci and less often coagulase-positive staphylococci or diphtheroids. The postoperative positive cultures in the gentamicin group were micrococci or *Proteus vulgaris* and were sensitive to gentamicin. Only after the use of sulfacetimide were antimicrobial-resistant organisms frequently found in the postoperative cultures.

No clinical differences and no postoperative infection were noted in any of the six categories; this is not unexpected, since the incidence of postoperative infection after cataract surgery is about 1:1,000.[5] In a study of clinical infection in decubitus ulcers, infection occurred only with bacterial populations in the 10^6 organisms per ml. range, well above any encountered in our studies.[6] However, one patient following cataract operation was thought clinically to have developed postoperative uveitis because of painless onset of hypopyon and vitreous haze occurring the seventh day after cataract extraction. The symptoms were associated with a rise in bacterial count—from 3,800 preoperatively to 10,000 postoperatively. The bacteria were micrococci and coagulase-positive staphylococci.

DISCUSSION

These results indicate that topical application of an antibiotic agent preoperatively and postoperatively is an effective prophylaxis against those postoperative infections that might be caused by the patient's own organisms entering the eye. This has been said to be the cause of the majority of postoperative infections.[7] This technique might not be as effective against a postoperative infection caused by a highly contaminated solution used for irrigating the operative field.[8] Nevertheless, since conjunctival cultures vary greatly from day to day[9] and since prolonged occlusion and antibiotic destruction of normal flora is required to produce an ecologic vacuum that fills up with pathogenic, antibiotic-resistant bacteria and fungi[10] short-term, intelligently directed antibiotic prophylaxis seems a reasonable measure in the immediate preoperative and postoperative period.[11]

Topical preoperative and postoperative use of gentamicin ointment or drops appears more effective in totally eliminating the external bacterial population than subconjunctival injection. However, since gentamicin given subconjunctivally at the time of surgery penetrates the eye in therapeutic levels,[12] this route of administration might be more effective in preventing infection from severe wound contamination at the time of surgery. Topical prophylactic ointment or drops might avoid the delayed infections associated with subconjunctival injection of antibiotics.[13, 14]

Gentamicin is an aminoglycoside bactericidal antibiotic, which is produced by *Micromonospora purpurea* and somewhat resembles neomycin, streptomycin, or kanamycin. It is a well-tolerated antibiotic that has a very wide spectrum of action against gram-positive as well as gram-negative organisms. It is particularly effective against *Pseudomonas.*[15] In studies at the Boston City Hospital it has been found to be the most generally effective antibiotic against gram-negative bacteria.[16] It was first released for systemic and dermatologic use and is now available for ophthalmic medication as a drop and ointment.

A potential advantage of gentamicin to the ophthalmologist is not only that it appears to be well-tolerated locally,[17] since we have recognized no toxic or allergic reaction in the already inflamed postoperative eye, but also that the drug can be ototoxic and nephrotoxic when given systemically. The recommended intramuscular dosage is 2 to 3 mg./Kg. Poor renal function increases the retention of gentamicin and causes more hazard of nephrotoxicity as well as ototoxicity, which can occur if blood levels exceed 13 to 15 μg./ml. If gentamicin is not used indiscriminately, ophthalmic bacteria may remain susceptible to it.

The technique described in this chapter appears to be a logical one for prospective study of antibiotic prophylaxis. It has the additional value of being able to evaluate quantitatively, in a human model and with a limited number of cases, the effectiveness of single antibiotics or drug mixtures. Because of the rarity of postcataract infection, it will be less effective in measuring possible incidence of this disaster. Retrospective study of postoperative infection requires many thousands of patients, possible only in a large city hospital, which might be less than ideally representative of our polluted environment. We plan to continue study of antibiotic prophylaxis before and after operation, to compare effectiveness of drugs, and to attain ideal methods of delivering medication.

REFERENCES

1. Allen, H. F., and Mangiaracine, A. B.: Bacterial endophthalmitis after cataract extraction, Arch. Ophthal. 72:454, 1964.

2. Locatcher-Khorazo, D., and Gutierrez, E.: Eye infections following cataract extraction, Amer. J. Ophthal. **41**:981, 1956.
3. Axenfeld, T.: The bacteriology of the eye, translated by A. MacNab, New York, 1908, William Wood & Co., p. 80.
4. Burns, R. P., Hansen, T., and others: An experimental model for evaluation of human conjunctivitis and topical antibiotic therapy, Canad. J. Ophthal. **3**:132, 1968.
5. Burns, R. P.: Postoperative infections in an ophthalmologic hospital, Amer. J. Ophthal. **48**:519, 1959.
6. Bendy, R. H., Jr., Nuccio, P. A., and others: Relationship of quantitative wound bacterial counts to healing of decubiti: effect of topical gentamicin, Antimicrobial Agents & Chemotherapy, 1964, p. 147 American Society for Microbiology.
7. Locatcher-Khorazo, D., Sullivan, N., and Gutierrez, E.: Staphylococcus aureus isolated from normal and infected eyes, Arch. Ophthal. **77**:370, 1967.
8. Ayliffe, G. A. J., and others: Postoperative infections with Pseudomonas aeruginosa in an eye hospital, Lancet **1**:1113, 1966.
9. Allansmith, M. R., Anderson, R. P., and Butterworth, M.: The meaning of preoperative cultures in ophthalmology, Trans. Amer. Acad. Ophthal. Otolaryng. **73**:683, 1969.
10. Marples, R. R., and Kligman, A. M.: Pyoderma due to Staphylococcus aureus following topical application of neomycin, J. Invest. Derm. **53**:11, 1969.
11. Polk, H. C., and Lopez-Mayor, J. R.: Postoperative wound infection: a prospective study of determinant factors and prevention, Surgery **66**:97, 1969.
12. Furgiuele, F. P.: Penetration of gentamicin into the aqueous humor of human Eyes, Amer. J. Ophthal. **69**:481, 1970.
13. Chalkley, T. H. F., and Shoch, D.: An evaluation of prophylactic subconjunctival antibiotic injection in cataract surgery, Amer. J. Ophthal. **64**:1084, 1967.
14. Aronstam, R. H.: Pitfalls of prophylaxis: alteration of postoperative infection by penicillin-streptomycin, Amer. J. Ophthal. **57**:312, 1964.
15. Burns, R. P.: Pseudomonas aeruginosa keratitis: mixed infections of the eye, Amer. J. Ophthal. **67**:257, 1969.
16. Sabath, L. N.: Drug resistance of bacteria, New Eng. J. Med. **280**:91, 1969.
17. Gordon, D. M.: Gentamicin sulfate in external eye infections, Amer. J. Ophthal. **69**:300, 1969.

Chapter 13

Problems in the use of antibiotics in ophthalmology

Irving H. Leopold, M.D.

New antimicrobials are found or synthesized each year and appear to enhance the ophthalmologist's armamentarium. However, it takes several years to evaluate the impact of new agents and the continued contribution of older ones. Constant reevaluation is mandatory since the benefits, as well as the untoward effects, of a new antimicrobial agent may not be known until several years after its clinical introduction.

The tremendous achievements in antiinfectious therapy in the past three decades have still left an important area of infectious ocular disease beyond our adequate control. Vision is still lost through ocular infection in spite of the vast number of chemotherapeutic and antibiotic substances available.

POSTOPERATIVE INFECTION

In general surgery, the severity of postoperative sepsis ranges from trivial, which is fairly common, to disastrous, which is rare.

Hospitals and the infection problem

A survey of infections developing at Johns Hopkins Hospital for 6 months in 1965 to 1966 on all services except psychiatry and dental surgery revealed a total of 592 detections, or an average of 100 per month, and an incidence among admissions of 4%.[1]

Wound infection developed in 2.3% of about 7,900 operations reviewed. About 9% of the operations accounted for over 36% of the infections; many of these operations were extensive. Gram-positive cocci and gram-negative bacilli were isolated from surgical wounds with nearly equal frequency. About one third of the patients were receiving antibiotics when infection developed. Penicillin and streptomycin were used most commonly.

Staphylococcus albus was isolated from 24% of wound infections in patients given prophylaxis and from 7.5% of infections in patients not given prophylaxis. In intraocular surgery, sepsis is always serious. In practically every intraocular infection, useful vision may be lost. In a series of 22 infections, evisceration of the eye was necessary in 11, and useful vision was lost in an additional seven.[2] In Birmingham, England, 15 intraocular infections led to the loss of six eyes.[3]

In considering intraocular infections, attention must be paid to possible infecting organisms, effective antiinfectious agents, and the proper dosage and route of administration of drugs in an effort to reduce the visual loss. In addition, a full knowledge of the potential toxicity of such antibiotic and chemotherapeutic antiinfectious agents must be kept in mind. In spite of these precautions, eyes are still lost to uncontrolled intraocular infection.

There are many reasons for this, some of which may defy our best efforts at the present time. The resistance of the patient—or lack of it—can often be the most important factor.

The pathogenic organism, particularly *Staphylococcus, Proteus,* and *Pseudomonas aeruginosa,* can vary in virulence, numbers, and resistance to therapeutic onslaught.

The host and his tissues vary in their ability to overcome infecting agents. Mutilated, necrotic tissue, poor blood supply, weak immunologic responses, and the presence of foreign bodies increase the chances of invasion and reduce the possibility of successful defense.

All ophthalmologists are aware of the necessity for using sterile solutions for ocular instillation. This can be ensured by means of heat or bacterial filters for heat-labile components. Most operating rooms in this country provide individual packaged solutions to be employed one for each patient. When this is done, it is unlikely to find the solution that was responsible for infection.

Preservatives

Any consideration of intraocular infection must note that at present there is no single ideal preservative for ophthalmic solutions. There are many preservatives that have been tried (Table 13-1). Each of these has some deficiency. The organic mecurials may produce deposits of mercury on the lens if used frequently.

Other means of preventing infection should be considered and have been stressed by many[4, 5] and most recently by Blowers[6] and Lowbury.[7] Among such areas are (1) skin disinfection, (2) cul-de-sac dis-

Table 13-1. Preservatives for ophthalmic solutions

Agent	*Evaluation*
Para-hydroxybenzoates	Effective when nearly saturated solution used Too irritant for normal use
Chlorocresol (0.05%)	Safe only for intact eye
Chlorobutanol (0.01%)	Effective but slow sterilizing agent
Organic mercurials (phenylmercuric nitrate)	Mercurialentis
Phenyl ethyl alcohol	Little value
Benzalkonium chloride (0.005%)	Effective—when properly handled
Polymyxin B sulfate	Effective when combined with anti-gram-positive agent
Chlorhexidine (Chlorhexide)	Effective—but incompatible with some ophthalmic agents

infection, (3) sterilization of instruments, and (4) preparation of the operating room staff and surgical team.

Skin disinfection

Disinfection of the skin can be carried out in several fashions. Lowbury, Lilly, and Bull[7, 8] recommended rubbing with an alcoholic solution of 0.5% chlorhexidine gluconate. For use on the patient's tissues this proves very satisfactory.

Cul-de-sac disinfection

Various antibiotics, singly or in combination, have been applied to the cul-de-sac for 24 to 48 hours preoperatively. This may reduce any susceptible existing bacterial flora. However, therapy in this fashion rarely sterilizes the cul-de-sac. If it does, the organism may reappear in a day or two after local therapy has ceased.

Cultures of the conjunctiva and margins before surgery may show no growth or reveal a pathogen. In the 24 to 48 hours after a swab is taken for culture, the cul-de-sac may be reinvaded. Local therapy with an antibiotic during the postculture, preoperative period may reduce this possibility. Special therapy against a revealed pathogen may reduce or eliminate the possibility of infection with such an organism.

Further work in the area of preoperative disinfection is needed, for there are objections to many of the presently available antibiotics. Bacitracin, chloramphenicol (Chloromycetin), neomycin, and polymyxin antibiotics are currently most popular. Objections to them are as follows:

1. Bacitracin fails to overcome some gram-positive organisms and does not act against gram-negative bacteria.
2. Chloramphenicol also fails to be effective against many strains. It is unlikely that blood dyscrasias will follow local therapy, but this possibility must be considered.

3. Neomycin is a frequent sensitizer, and although it has a broad spectrum, neomycin-resistant staphylococci do occur.
4. Polymyxin fails to overcome gram-positive organisms, as well as some gram-negative organisms. Therefore it must be combined with agents active in the latter areas.

Studies are beginning to appear with newer antibiotics: gentamicin (Garamycin), cephaloridine (Keflordin), cephalothin (Keflin), carbenicillin (Pyopen), and various quaternary ammonium compounds alone or in combination with polymyxin. Antiseptics are preferable to antibiotics because of their wide range of activity against organisms and the avoidance of stimulating possible emergence of antibiotic-resistant strains. The routine use of an antiseptic preparation prophylactically for several days preoperatively might overcome the need for conjunctival cultures.

The value of cul-de-sac cultures preoperatively has been studied many times, most recently by Nolan.[9] Conjunctival and nasal cultures were taken on admission from patients entering for cataract extraction. Cultures were repeated immediately before operation. Some pathogenic organisms noted on admission had disappeared at time of surgery. Conversely, pathogenic organisms not present on admission were sometimes found immediately before surgery. Uncomplicated extractions were done in the presence of pathogenic organisms, but infection did occur where a pathogen was present.

It is evident that cultures taken 48 hours prior to surgery are inadequate as a safety measure. Perhaps the routine use of antiseptic solutions will reduce the number of pathogens and of resultant intraocular infections.

Nasal cultures taken by Nolan did not show any correlation with conjunctival findings or with subsequent operative results. Thus, Nolan stated that the nasal flora does not appear to be a significant guide to likely conjunctival pathogens and can be ignored for intraocular operations.

Attempts to sterilize the cul-de-sac with antiseptics or antibiotics are not always successful, although a reduction in flora does usually occur. Studies at The Mount Sinai Hospital indicate that pathogens can appear occasionally in eyes pretreated with quaternary ammonium compounds combined with polymyxin and that, rarely, staphylococci resistant to neomycin and to chloramphenicol appear. Further search for effective means of sterilizing the cul-de-sac is indicated.

Incidence of intraocular infection

The incidence of intraocular infection after surgery varies.

It is important to realize that the range of sepsis from one institution to another can be determined by many factors. There must be both a loophole in technique and an opportunistic organism with the necessary characteristics to permit it to penetrate the loophole. One institution with a low incidence of infections and another with a high incidence may have the same techniques and same loophole. However, the latter institution has been visited by the effective opportunistic organism and the other has not. A long period of freedom from infection need not mean that no loopholes exist.

At one institution, 40 cases of endophthalmitis were encountered in 8,277 cataract extractions over a period of 12 years—1953 to 1964.[10] There were 40 infections in the 5 recently reported outbreaks in England, covering a period of less than 2 years, and decidedly fewer operations.

Dramatic outbreaks of infections are usually caused by *Pseudomonas aeruginosa* from contaminated solutions, as occurred in England. Sporadic postoperative infections are most often associated with *Staphylococcus aureus.* These can come from the patient, the operating room environment, or the surgical team.

Blowers,[6] in summarizing the areas that require attention if one is to reduce infection after ocular surgery, included the following:

1. Modern ventilation in the operating rooms and in areas where instruments are sterilized and operating trays are prepared
2. Preparation and movements of the operating team

Sterilization of instruments

Heat, dry or by steam, is the one safe method for sterilizing sharp and other instruments for ophthalmic operations.

Preparation and movements of the operating team

Shedding of organisms by the surgical staff is a distinct possibility. This possibility is increased if one of the members has a septic focus and if there is much movement. Regular bathing, particularly with hexachlorophene-containing soap, reduces skin carriage of organisms such as staphylococci; but shower baths should not be taken immediately before an operation. Such a procedure appears to increase the number of staphylcocci shed.

Preoperative scrubbing does reduce the number of available bacteria but does not eliminate them. The risk of infection from the hands can be reduced to the lowest level only by wearing rubber gloves.

There is less dispersal of organisms from the operating team if the operating gowns are closed at the trouser apertures and if the gowns are made of closely woven, waterproof fabric.

Table 13-2. Specific toxicity of antimicrobial agents

Antimicrobial agent	*Possible toxicity*
Penicillin	Severe hypersensitivity
Methicillin (Staphcillin)	Nephritis, leukopenia (bone marrow depression), pain at injection site, hypersensitivity
Oxacillin (Prostaphlin)	Same as methicillin
Nafcillin (Unipen)	Same as methicillin
Cloxacillin (TegoPen)	Same as methicillin
Streptomycin	Vertigo, tinnitus, deafness
Kanamycin (Kantrex)	Eighth cranial nerve damage, renal damage
Colistin (Coly-Mycin)	Renal damage
Tetracycline	Superinfection, gastrointestinal symptoms
Chloramphenicol (Chloromycetin)	Bone marrow depression
Erythromycin (Erythrocin)	Hypersensitivity (rare), gastrointestinal disturbance
Novobiocin (Albamycin sodium)	Leukopenia (mild), skin pigmentation, rashes, hypersensitivity
Bacitracin	Renal irritation
Vancomycin (Vancocin)	Eighth nerve damage, renal irritation, phlebitis, hypersensitivity
Polymyxin B	Renal damage, paresthesia, vertigo (mild)
Isoniazid	Peripheral neuritis
Para-aminosalicylic acid	Gastritis
Cycloserine (Seromycin)	Central nervous system irritation
Viomycin (Vinactane)	Eighth nerve damage, renal damage
Sulfonamides	Neutropenia (bone marrow), fever, dermatitis, renal effects, hypersensitivity
Cephalosporin	Hypersensitivity, leukopenia, pain at injection site
Lincomycin (Lincocin)	Diarrhea, myalgia
Amphotericin (Fungizone)	Renal damage, fever, phlebitis, hypersensitivity, hypokalemia, anemia

TOXICITY OF CHEMOTHERAPEUTIC AND ANTIBIOTIC SUBSTANCES

Toxic features may be divided into two types: those that are local and peculiar to the ocular structures and those that are systemic. Those that are local and peculiar to the ocular structures usually follow local administration of the antibiotic or chemotherapeutic substance. These include the following:

1. Hypersensitivity
2. Local irritative or necrotic action
3. Alteration of the local bacterial flora, allowing replacement flora or development of locally pathogenic strains as well as resistant ones

Systemic and life-threatening reactions to antibiotics include the following:

1. Shock
2. Superinfection (primary resistant staphylococci)

3. Severe skin reactions, exfoliative dermatitis, or erythema multiforme (anaphylactoid purpura)
4. Blood dyscrasias—for example, aplastic anemia
5. Angioneurotic edema
6. Respiratory tract involvement

In addition, the following may be considered as diseases induced by antibiotics and chemotherapeutic agents:

1. Disease caused by resistant staphylococci—septicemia, endocarditis, pseudomembranous enterocolitis, diarrhea, and pneumonia
2. Gram-negative bacteremia as well as moniliasis (superinfection)
3. Mucous membrane syndrome—deficiency in vitamin K and vitamin B complex
4. Neurologic disorders—for example, peripheral neuritis, tinnitus, and vertigo
5. Serum sickness—angioneurotic edema, skin reactions, anaphylactoid shock, and photosensitivity
6. Blood dyscrasias
7. Gray syndrome of infants

It is apparent that all antibiotics (Table 13-2) may arouse toxic effects or allergic reactions. Some of them are minor, but occasionally they can be life-threatening and even lethal.

USAGE AND SPECIFIC TOXIC EFFECTS

The importance of adverse reactions to drugs is obvious in clinical practice. Yet few definite facts are known about them, and even their incidence is not accurately established. It has been estimated that between 5% and 10% of patients admitted to hospitals experience some toxic reaction to drugs. However, recent investigations into the incidence of adverse reactions to drugs in the hospital were carried out at the Dermatology Department of the Royal Free Hospital in London and suggest that the true figure is much lower. It may be that the lower figure in the study reported by Sarconi[11] is because of the fact that each case was scrutinized in detail by several people, rather than the usual method of reporting in which reports of drug reactions are noted and accepted as such, but are probably not drug-induced reactions.

In a total of 1,846 patients admitted as inpatients over a 2-month period, 45 adverse reactions were observed. Of these, two were considered to be proved, one from ampicillin and one from cloxacillin. Nineteen others were considered clinically definite. There were 13 probable cases. Eleven were considered doubtful. This represented a total incidence of 2.4% of all admissions.

There is no doubt that antibiotics head the list, as in other series that have been reported. It is evident from this study that ampicillin may be a frequent offender. Usually a rash appears in 5 to 14 days after starting treatment. The rash is mainly papular in nature, bright red in color, and appears predominantly over the extensor aspects of the legs and the trunk, with marked concentration in the region of the elbows and knees, thus resembling the distribution of erythema multiforme.

The doctor in clinical practice is well aware of the necessity for distinguishing between an allergic reaction and a toxic manifestation. The cause of the manifestation will determine whether he will be able to continue administration and whether the drug can ever be used by that patient in the future. All unwanted effects caused by drugs are by no means hypersensitive reactions. We know that harmful effects of drugs may be caused by intolerance or idiosyncrasy based on some enzymatic defects in the blood or tissue cells. Only a relatively small proportion of cutaneous eruptions, thrombocytic purpura, bone marrow aplasia, and certain forms of jaundice are based on true hypersensitivity, that is, on the effects of antigen-antibody interreaction. No doubt new forms of enzymatic and metabolic abnormalities will be discovered as causes of reactions to drugs.

Each of these antibiotics has a specific type of toxicity. In some, such as the newer penicillins, experience has not been great, and other toxic features may become apparent as the agents are employed over the ensuing years. Penicillin has produced the greatest number and most severe reactions of all the antibiotics available. These have been largely the hypersensitivity type of reaction.

The tetracyclines appear to have produced the most cases of superinfections.

Bone marrow depression has been most common with chloramphenicol, of all the antibiotic substances, but this has been quite infrequent.

Side effects cannot always be avoided. However, steps can be taken to minimize them. Hypersensitivity reactions can be eliminated to some extent by prior skin testing or by the use of the Shelley basophilic degranulation test. By weaning the patient from the drug as soon as the condition allows, one can often reduce the incidence of side effects. Large systemic dosage as well as large doses given subconjunctivally may often have to be used with these agents in order to control intraocular infection. This means the patient is threatened with toxic side effects. However, because the agents generally are used only for a few days, the chance of appearance of the undesirable activities may be reduced.

Much information concerning hypersensitivity reactions has been acquired over the years. Patients who have shown hypersensitivity to local sulfonamide therapy may develop extremely severe reactions to subsequent oral administration. Reactions are less likely to occur if treatment is confined to a few days and are less frequent if sulfonamides are applied in the form of a thick paste or miscible cream rather than as a powder.

Patients with reactions to locally applied sulfonamides will usually respond to a simple patch test in which a 50% sulfonamide powder in hydrous lanolin (Lamo) is applied to the skin after light scarification. Subjects who develop hypersensitivity reactions to systemic sulfonamides usually fail to respond to skin tests, but they show an immediate allergic reaction when tested by intradermal injection of serum from a patient receiving the appropriate sulfonamide. For a positive result, the test serum must contain at least 2 mg./100 ml. and should come from a patient who has been taking sulfonamides for at least 5 days.

Sometimes the sensitivities are specific for a particular sulfonamide. On other occasions, particularly after local therapy, the patients react to all sulfonamides and also to the common radical, sulfanilic acid. They may also show reactions to procaine, which possesses the same aminophenyl radical.

Patients can sometimes be desensitized by a week's course of increasing oral doses twice daily, starting with 0.1 gm.

Hypersensitivity to penicillin presents a far more serious problem than that to any other antibiotic. The intital contact may be hidden. Usually two types of reactions are seen: (1) urticaria and fever and (2) immediate profound shock that may be fatal in a few minutes. The latter most often follows injection, but it may take place after oral or local application, or after a minute dose, such as a test for sensitivity.

To avoid hypersensitivity reactions one must take a careful history of previous reactions. Routine sensitivity tests show only the less dangerous type of hypersensitivity. Patients with asthma and other known sensitivities are exceptional risks and should be given other antibiotics. Penicillin should be used only when there is ample justification.

DeWeck[12] suggested using penicilloyl-polypeptide compound for skin testing, as he believes the actual hapten responsible for the sensitivity is not the penicillin-protein combination, but penicillinic acid or a penicilloyl derivative of it. This substance is slowly formed from penicillin in solution. Penicillinic acid can induce sensitivity, but the penicilloyl-polypeptide compound does not induce hypersensitivity, although it can detect it.

Definite tests have been devised to assess the sensitivity of patients to penicillin. These may be classified as skin tests, serologic tests, and tests of histamine release.

Skin testing

Crystalline benzo-penicillin solutions have been used in the oldest and simplest of the techniques for skin testing. Unfortunately, they have little value. False-positive and false-negative reactions occur with frequency. Anaphylactic reactions, including at least one fatal reaction, have been reported after the intradermal injection of minute amounts of penicillin.[13] The same comments apply to conjunctival testing.

A suitable perparation for skin testing should allow one to assess the individual status of sensitivity correctly without itself sensitizing or producing a hypersensitivity reaction.[14] Such a substance, penicilloyl-polylysine, has been synthesized. It was hoped that this substance would overcome all the disadvantages inherent in the use of penicillin itself. Penicilloyl-polylysine is not sensitizing. Repeated skin testing has failed to produce antibodies in experimental animals. There is no record of a reaction having occurred in a human being as a result of testing with it. Its effectiveness in screening patients for hypersensitivity is, however, currently under question. There are individuals who have hypersensitivity to penicillin who fail to react to penicilloyl-polylysine. Others may exhibit a strongly positive skin test to penicilloyl-polylysine, yet experience no clinical reaction following penicillin treatment. It appears that benzo-penicillin is a more effective detector of potential immediate reactors than is penicilloyl-polylysine.[15, 16] If one carries out the tests with both reagents, penicillyol-polylysine and benzo-penicillin, a strongly positive reaction increases the chances that an immediate reaction following penicillin treatment will occur.

A negative reaction to both materials would indicate that an immediate reaction following administration of penicillin would not occur, but this view is based on only a relatively small number of cases. In addition, a negative reaction does not rule out the occurrence of a late urticarial or serum sickness type of reaction.

Serologic testing

Red blood cells preincubated with benzo-penicillin sometimes will be agglutinated by human serum. The antibodies detected by this technique are specific. Usually low titers have been obtained. If one preincubates a red cell with benzo-penicillin at an alkaline pH, the sensitivity of the test is increased. However, no correlation has been found between the titer obtained and the level of hypersensitivity as estimated by skin reaction to penicilloyl-polylysine. The high titers persist for only a few weeks after an allergic reaction. This feature also tends to limit the usefulness of the test. Although the test can be used in confirming a diagnosis of penicillin hypersensitivity, it is not suitable for determining routinely whether or not a patient lacking a history of previous reactions will react to the administration of penicillin.[12]

Histamine-release testing

A histamine-release test is based on the release of histamine from cells other than mast cells—mainly from the basophils. The assumption has been made that, during the reaction between antigen and antibody, the granules of living basophils release histamine, and visible changes occur in the cell.[17] The test can be modified in several ways. One can use the patient's own blood as a source of basophils or, if basophils are scarce, one can use rabbit leukocytes. Benzo-penicillin has been used as the antigen.

In general, the high proportion of positive results has been observed in patients with a history of reaction less than 2 years previously. If a longer period has elapsed since the reaction, results are more variable; in the temporary anergic state following a severe reaction, results of the test have been negative. The test has been criticized on the grounds that the results depend largely on the personal judgment of the technologist observing subtle alterations in the cytologic characteristics of the basophils. In addition, serum controls may contain several abnormal cells, making interpretation of the test difficult.[18, 19] The test may be modified so that both serum control and serum penicillin sample are applied to the same slide, making it easier to compare the cytologic characteristics of the test basophils,[19] and one may attempt to remove the personal bias of the observer by measuring fluorometrically the amount of histamine released from a system containing benzo-penicillin and rabbit blood possibly sensitized with fresh human serum.

Lymphocyte transformation test

There is no problem in the field of immunology that appears more urgent than the development of a relatively simple and reliable in vitro technique for the diagnosis of drug hypersensitivity. Halpern and Amache[20] described a lymphocyte transformation test in which a significant number of blood lymphocytes are transformed into blast cells when lymphocytes from sensitive individuals are cultured in the presence of specific antigen. Tests are considered positive if more than 4% blast cells occur after 4 days of culture in the presence of antigen, provided the control cultures without antigen from the same patient and the control cultures with the same antigen and lymphocytes from normal individuals contain less than 2% blast cells. The test has been evaluated for penicillin, various other antibiotics, insulin, acetylsalicylic acid, and local anesthetics. The test has been positive whether the allergy was of the immediate or delayed type. Corticotherapy or addition of steroids to the culture media inhibited the specific lymphoblastic transformation.

Blood dyscrasias

The most serious complication of sulfonamide therapy is damage to blood-forming organs. Anemia, purpura, and agranulocytosis may result.

Therapy can follow a short course, but in the majority of cases it involves a prolonged schedule of high dosage. Hypersensitivity may be a factor.

Agranulocytosis commonly develops within 2 to 3 weeks after the onset of therapy. Fever is often the first sign. The presence of fever at this time should be a warning.

Chloramphenicol is a potentially dangerous bone marrow depressant. Granulocytopenia is uncommon. Purpura and pallor are the first signs. Blood counts show a deficiency of all blood cells. Death is the usual outcome despite transfusions. This complication may appear during the months after cessation of therapy. There seems to be no absolutely safe dosage schedule.

Repeated blood counts can be a safeguard. A diminished reticulocyte count is the earliest sign; at this stage the disease is reversible. This test is as accurate as a bone marrow biopsy. It is advisable to repeat this test every 2 days.

Gastrointestinal disturbance

The tetracyclines are the chief offenders of the antibiotics to the gastrointestinal tract. Some of the effects may be caused by irritation, but they are most probably caused by superinfection. Three kinds of organisms fill the void left by the flora inhibition induced by these broad-spectrum agents. *Candida albicans* may proliferate in the mouth, pharynx, and bowel. *Proteus* and *Pseudomonas* species resistant to the tetracyclines may become predominant in the bowel. A resistant strain of *Staphylococcus aureus* may be responsible for a serious superinfection. Diarrhea is the outstanding symptom and should be a stimulus for the search of fecal films for positive stains of the offending organisms.

It is doubtful that vitamin B deficiency is an important factor in this gastrointestinal disturbance. It is also doubtful that one tetracycline is less damaging in this regard than another.

Effect of antibiotics on the gastrointestinal tract[21]

Antimicrobial agents appear to have two general types of effects on the gastrointestinal tract:

1. Alterations of the bacterial population
2. Direct toxic effects related to the pharmacologic properties of the agent independent of microbial activity

Alteration of the bacterial flora may lead to staphylococcic enterocolitis or candidiasis and can produce disturbances of nutrition, growth, resistance to infection, and selection of more resistant strains.

The nonmicrobial effects may include histaminic release by the polymyxins, staining of teeth by tetracycline, gastrointestinal upset by tetracycline, ampicillin, lincomycin hydrochloride, liver diseases by tetracycline, neonatal jaundice by novobiocin, and allergic cholestatic jaundice by erythromycin estolate.

Liver disease

Erythromycin and oleandomycin (Matromycin) can produce mild gastrointestinal disturbances, but more threatening is the potential for liver damage. Usually abdominal pain, fever, hepatic enlargement, and increase in bilirubin indicate the hepatic involvement. All disturbances clear as the drugs are withdrawn.

Eighth nerve damage

Defects of hearing, ranging from decrease in auditory acuity to complete deafness, may be noted with vancomycin, kanamycin, neomycin, and gentamicin. This eighth nerve involvement appears to be related to dosage schedule, duration of therapy, and renal efficiency. However, deafness has been reported with small doses, particularly in the presence of impaired renal function. If the kidneys are impaired, it is best to use some other agent, such as methicillin or oxacillin, for resistant staphylococci.

The most serious effects of streptomycin are vestibular disturbance and deafness with dihydrostreptomycin. Although chances of such side effects are related to total dosage, renal impairment and age in excess of 40 years increase the risk.

The severity of the threat to vision by a properly diagnosed ocular infection is a criterion for the use of these agents in spite of their toxicity.

Thrombophlebitis

The most common complication of vancomycin and amphotericin B therapy is thrombophlebitis at the injection site. In order to minimize this, the antibiotic must be diluted adequately and given slowly, with leakage avoided and different veins employed for each new injection. The dilution may be in normal saline or a 5% dextrose solution. The concentration should not exceed 1%, and the rate of injection should be 2 ml./min.

Renal toxicity

A number of antibiotics may produce renal damage. In this group are neomycin, kanamycin, polymyxin, colistin, amphotericin, and methicillin. The change in the renal tubules is usually reversible, but permanent damage can occur. Amphotericin has been shown to produce changes in glomeruli as well. These agents should be avoided in patients with impaired renal function. In those in whom the drugs are employed, urinalyses, blood urea nitrogen, and other tests of renal insufficiency should be performed regularly.

Sulfonamide renal reactions can produce ureteral colic, dysuria, flank tenderness, and oliguria. Crystals may be found in the urine. Gentle irrigation of the ureters with 10% sodium bicarbonate solution should result in immediate and adequate urine flow. Sulfonamides can damage the kidney by sensitivity reaction affecting the glomeruli, tubular degeneration, obstruction, and the effects of intravascular hemolysis. Alkalinization of the urine by concomitant administration of sodium bicarbonate and potassium citrate may reduce the incidence of sulfonamide crystals.

Route of administration

For external infections, the ophthalmologist is well aware that he can apply the medication in the form of drops, ointments, cotton packs, and lamellae, or wafers. Iontophoresis, corneal baths, and subconjunctival injections can be used. Drugs can also be given locally by intracameral injection.

Systemically, drugs can be administered orally, intramuscularly, or intravenously. Oral administration, with rare exceptions, demands large dosage schedules—much greater than those usually employed in general medicine.

Not all agents penetrate equally well into intraocular tissues and fluids. Many agents that fail to penetrate into the normal eye will penetrate into the inflamed eye, because the blood–aqueous barrier is decreased in the presence of the inflammatory process. It is essential, however, that the ophthalmologist be aware of the ability of the agent he is employing to penetrate from the bloodstream into the eye and to the area of the infected tissue.

AGENTS AVAILABLE

The agents available for the control of intraocular infection or ocular infection are listed in Tables 13-3 to 13-5, with suggested dosage schedules. They are also listed according to the organisms that are most often susceptible to each agent. Only a few agents have been added in recent years. Special mention should be made of the newer penicillins. Streptococcal and pneumococcal infections continue to be responsive to the original and commonly employed penicillin G. However, the incidence of staphylococcal infection resistant to penicillin has increased since the 1940's, and it is likely that many of our intraocular infections are caused by penicillin-resistant staphylococci. Therefore, attention must be paid to the new semisynthetic penicillins prepared by changing the side chains of 6-aminopenicillinic acid (6-APA). This is the basic penicillin nucleus.

Penicillin G is still the best drug for infections caused by nonpenicillinase-producing staphylococci, streptococci, pneumococci, gonococci,

Table 13-3. Dosage for systemic therapy in intraocular infection

Agent	*Dosage*
Agents effective against gram-positive and gram-negative organisms	
Ampicillin (Penbritin)	2 gm. priming dose, orally, I.M., I.V., and 1 gm. every 6 hours
Carbenicillin (Pyopen)	5 to 7 gm. every 4 hours, I.V.
Penicillin with streptomycin	(*see* Agents effective against gram-positive infections)
	1 gm. priming dose, I.M., and 0.5 gm. every 8 hours
Cephalothin (Keflin)	2 gm. every 4 hours, I.M.
Cephalexin (Keflex)	2 gm. priming dose, orally, and 1 gm. every 8 hours
Cephaloridine (Loridine)	2 gm. priming dose, I.M., and 1 gm. every 8 hours
Chloramphenicol (Chloromycetin)	3 gm. priming dose, orally, I.M., I.V., and 1 gm. every 8 hours
Gentamicin (Garamycin)	1 mg./kg. every 8 hours, I.M.
Kanamycin (Kantrex)	0.5 gm. every 8 hours, I.M.
Sulfadiazine (Cremodiazine)	2 gm. priming dose, orally, I.V., and 1 gm. every 6 hours
Tetracycline	1 gm. priming dose, orally, I.M., I.V., and 0.5 gm. every 8 hours
Agents effective against gram-positive infections	
Erythromycin (Erythrocin)	
propionate (Ilosone)	1 gm. priming dose, orally, and 0.5 gm. every 6 hours
succinate	100 mg. every 4 hours, I.V.
lactobionate	250 to 500 mg. every 4 hours, I.V.
Lincomycin (Lincocin)	2 gm. priming dose, orally, and 1 gm. every 6 hours
	1 gm., I.M., initially and 600 mg. every 8 hours
	600 mg., I.V., every 8 hours
Methicillin (Staphcillin) (for penicillinase-producing bacteria)	4 gm. every 6 hours, I.M.
Oxacillin (sodium oxacillin) (Prostaphlin) (for penicillinase-producing bacteria)	2 gm. every 6 hours, I.M., I.V.
Penicillin G (aqueous) (for nonpenicillinase-producing bacteria)	20 million units daily, interrupted or continuous I.V. infusion
Novobiocin (Albamycin)	0.5 gm. every 6 hours, orally, and 0.5 mg. every 12 hours, I.M., I.V.
Vancomycin (Vancocin)	2 gm. priming dose, I.V., and 1 gm. every 12 hours I.V.
Agent effective against fungi	
Amphotericin B (Fungizone)	0.25 to 1.5 mg./kg., I.V.

Table 13-4. Dosage for subconjunctival therapy in intraocular infections

Agent	*Dosage*
Bacitracin	10,000 units
with polymyxin B	10 mg. (1 mg. = 10,000 units)
or colistin (Coly-Mycin)	15 mg.
Cephalothin (Keflin)	50 mg.
Cephaloridine (Loridine)	25 to 50 mg.
Chloramphenicol (Chloromycetin)	1.25 mg.
0.7 ml. of 15%	
suspension of micronized material, sodium	
succinate	100 mg.
Erythromycin	2.5 mg.
(lactobionate) (Erythrocin)	up to 50 mg.
or novobiocin with polymyxin B	10 mg. (1 mg. = 10,000 units)
Gentamicin (Garamycin)	1.25 to 2.5 mg.
Kanamycin (Kantrex)	10 to 20 mg.
Lincomycin (Lincocin)	50 to 75 mg.
Neomycin	100 to 500 mg.
Penicillin G	500,000 to 1 million units
or methicillin (Staphcillin)	150 mg.
with streptomycin	50 mg.
Tetracycline	2.5 to 5 mg.

Table 13-5. Solutions for intracameral injection or irrigation

Agent	*Dosage*
Bacitracin	500 to 1,000 units
Chloramphenicol (Chloromycetin)	1 to 2 mg.
Colistin (Coly-Mycin)	0.1 mg.
Erythrocycin (Erythrocin)	1 to 2 mg.
Methicillin (Staphcillin)	1 mg.
Neomycin	2.5 mg.
Penicillin G	1,000 to 4,000 units
Polymyxin B	0.1 mg.
Streptomycin	0.5 to 5 mg.
Tetracycline	2.5 to 5 mg.

and clostridia. There is no drug that compares with its effectiveness, lack of toxicity, and economy.

There are many agents that can control infection caused by a specific organism. However, experience has indicated that for each organism there is usually one drug (rarely a combination of drugs) that is more likely to be effective than another agent or a combination of agents.

When the patient cannot tolerate the first choice or fails to respond, there is a choice of alternate drugs available.

The newer, semisynthetic penicillins fall into three groups: (1) acid-resistant penicillins, (2) penicillinase-resistant penicillins, and (3) broad-spectrum penicillins.

The acid-resistant penicillins consist of phenethicillin (Chemipen), propicillin (Brocillin), and phenbenicillin (Penspek). The main advantage of this group of penicillins over penicillin G is the resistance to gastric acid degradation: thus, high levels of the drug can be obtained rapidly after oral administration.* Subconjunctival injections have caused violent tissue reactions. Parenteral forms of these drugs are not available at present for human use. The acid-resistant penicillins are of little value to the ophthalmologist at the present time, for they are given orally and do not produce the high blood level favorable for ocular penetration.

Other derivatives, such as methicillin, oxacillin, cloxacillin, diphenicillin (Ancillin), and nafcillin, are resistant to hydrolysis by penicillinase. Methicillin, oxacillin, and nafcillin are available in the United States. Of these, oxacillin may be given orally. It appears to produce definite serum levels that may penetrate into the eye. However, careful laboratory control is necessary, if oxacillin is used orally, to ascertain that it has been absorbed and can be effective. The greatest experience to date has been with methicillin. This may be given intramuscularly or intravenously. It penetrates poorly into the normal eye but will penetrate past the blood–aqueous barrier in the inflamed eye. It is similar to penicillin in penetration. All of the agents are bound in the serum, so that not all of them detectable in the serum are free to pass across the blood–aqueous barrier. Methicillin and ampicillin have been found to be the least serum-bound of the newer penicillins.

Ampicillin is the first available semisynthetic penicillin that is effective against gram-negative bacteria. Chemically, it is alpha-aminobenzyl penicillin. It is active against some strains of *Escherichia coli, Shigella* and *Salmonella.* It seems to be equivalent in the strains tested to the action of tetracycline and chloramphenicol. It is quite active against *Hemophilus influenzae.* It is not effective against many strains of *Pseudomonas,* nor is it very effective against nonpenicillinase-producing staphylococci and gram-negative bacteria such as some *Escherichia coli* and *Proteus* bacilli, which may also elaborate the enzyme. A parenteral preparation is available; it is also given orally. Studies in our laboratory to date have shown that this drug penetrates adequately into the normal experimental animal and human eye. It passes readily into the inflamed eye. It is unlikely, because of its lack of effect against penicillinase-producing staphylococci, that it will be of great therapeutic value to ophthalmologists, in spite of its penetration performance. However, its ease of penetration makes it potentially useful for combined therapy.

---

*Duer and Maas found that phenethicillin given intramuscularly to normal rabbits reached the aqueous but not the vitreous.

EFFECTS OF THE NEWER DRUGS

Penicillins

Organisms develop resistance to the newer penicillins, and superinfections by fungi as well as by gram-negative bacilli have already been reported. Each of these has the possibility of producing hypersensitivity reactions in the recipient, and there may be a crossed allergic reaction in people who are sensitive to penicillin G, although this does not always occur. Bone marrow depressions have also been reported in a few patients during methicillin therapy, so that blood counts must be performed routinely. An elevation of serum glutamic oxaloacetic transaminase (SGOT) has been noted in an occasional patient being treated with oxacillin and ampicillin.

The synthetic penicillins have once again brought serious staphylococcal infections within therapeutic range. This type of infection must still be anticipated, particularly when serious staphylococcal infections supervene in settings wherein host offenses are seriously compromised by underlying disease and therapy.

The present status of the new penicillins may be summarized as follows: penicillins are bactericidal, essentially nontoxic, and available for peroral or parenteral use. They possess antibacterial spectra that include almost all of the common pathogens. Their chief disadvantages are a propensity to cause allergic hypersensitivity reactions.

Methicillin

Methicillin (Staphcillin) is the agent of choice in the treatment of severe penicillin G resistant staphylococcal infections. It is administered parenterally and is therefore limited almost exclusively to hospital usage. Methicillin is used in combination with penicillin G for the initial treatment of severe staphylococcal infections until the resistance pattern of the infecting strain can be determined. Methicillin may be considered for preoperative prophylaxis when staphylococcal infections are common and when such infections present intolerable hazards as in ophthalmology. It shares crossed allergic hypersensitivity reactions with the other penicillins and has caused a few well-documented cases of reversible bone marrow depression and of nephropathy. It is important that clinicians recognize nephropathy as an untoward effect of methicillin because of its potential danger to renal function if the drug is not discontinued.[22] Resistance to methicillin is beginning to appear in the United States just as resistance has been reported on the European continent.[23, 24]

Oxacillin

Oxacillin (Prostaphlin) may be used for the treatment of moderately severe infections caused by penicillin G–resistant staphylococci. It is suitable for oral administration, preferably on an empty stomach. Oxacillin may be used to complete a course of therapy initiated with methicillin. It may be used to treat mixed staphylococcal-streptococcal infection after penicillin G has failed. Parenterally, oxacillin may be used to treat severe penicillin G resistance to staphylococcal infections, although experience with oxacillin is not as extensive as with methicillin. Oxacillin also shares the allergenic hazards of penicillin and has caused transient elevations of SGOT activity.

Cloxacillin

Cloxacillin (TegoPen), which is still undergoing clinical trials in the United States, yields somewhat higher and more predictable serum concentrations than does oxacillin, to which it is closely related chemically. Should these preliminary results be widely confirmed, cloxacillin will probably replace oxacillin in clinical usage.

Currently available tests for determining whether a person will react allergically to penicillin are inadequate, and the question of whether a person allergic to one penicillin will also be allergic to other penicillins cannot be answered with certainty. These problems, coupled with data on the immunologic distinction between penicillins, indicate that allergic reactions are too complex to be defined by a single test. It is concluded that, at present, administrations of penicillin must be based on the physician's judgment and on the case history.

Choice of penicillinase-resistant semisynthetic penicillin

In vitro testing studies indicate that milligram for milligram nafcillin and oxacillin are about four times as active as methicillin against strains of penicillinase-producing *Staphylococcus aureus.*

The protein binding of methicillin is only about 40% as compared to approximately 90% for nafcillin and 95% for oxacillin.

The differences in activity and protein binding influence the recommended doses. These range for methicillin from 6 to 24 grains per day for an adult, and from 3 to 12 gm. for nafcillin and oxacillin. As summarized in *Medical Letter*, April 18, 1969, vol. 2, there is no evidence that the three drugs differ in effectiveness when the recommended doses are used.

The pH of the solutions used for intravenous administration must be watched to preserve activity and prevent flocculation.

Medical Letter also noted that methicillin has been associated with reversible nephritis, but no such association has been reported with oxacillin and nafcillin.

All three solutions are formulated as sodium salts. This must be appreciated in patients who might be adversely affected by large sodium intake.

It has been suggested that penicillinase-resistant pencillins be used to increase the susceptibility of gram-negative bacteria to antibiotics.

Many gram-negative bacteria elaborate beta-lactamases capable of inactivating penicillin and related antibiotics. Certin semisynthetic penicillins like methicillin, while not very active against these microbes, are very slowly destroyed by these enzymes of the gram-negative bacteria but have high binding affinity for them. This suggests the possibility of using a penicillinase-resistant semisynthetic penicillin combined with a hydrolyzable penicillin or cephalosporin to protect the latter from the action of penicillinase and thereby increase its antibacterial effectiveness.[25]

In vitro studies were made of 100 strains of gram-negative bacilli isolated from blood or urine in patients with clinical infection who were found to be resistant to at least 50 μg. ampicillin or cephalothin, or both. The organisms included 30 strains of *Escherichia coli,* 31 of *Klebsiella*-aerobacter group, 8 of indole-positive *Proteus,* and 31 of *Pseudomonas aeruginosa.* Sensitivity testing was carried out in trypticase soy broth. Benzyl penicillin, ampicillin, and cephalothin were used as antibiotics, and methicillin, nafcillin, and oxacillin as inhibitors.

The combination of cephalothin and oxacillin was effective against the twelve strains of *Klebsiella*-aerobacter organisms tested. A positive interaction was observed with at least one combination of antibiotic and inhibitor in 81% of cells or strains.

With *E. coli,* no one combination was consistently effective against all strains, but at least one combination was consistently effective against 83% of the strains tested.

Nafcillin was effective against *Pseudomonas,* inhibiting 4 strains alone and the other 27 with an additional antibiotic. An effective combination was found for 6 of the 8 indole-positive *Proteus* organisms. In all, an effective combination was found for 86 of the 100 strains studied.

With the strains of the *Klebsiella*-aerobacter group and of *E. coli,* evidence was found that the effects were actually synergistic. The effects with *Pseudomonas aeruginosa* seemed to be additive and related to a significant degree to the antibacterial activity of nafcillin.

This approach has not been tried, knowingly, for ophthalmologic infection, but it is well reasoned and merits a trial.

Carbenicillin

Carbenicillin (Pyopen) is a new semisynthetic penicillin having a wide antibacterial range of activity against gram-positive and gram-negative pathogens. This antibacterial spectrum of activity is similar to ampicillin, except that carbenicillin provides significant activity against most strains of *Pseudomonas pyocyanea,* indole-positive *Proteus* species, and some strains of Enterobacter not susceptible to ampicillin. Carbenicillin is bactericidal, unstable to staphylococcal penicillinase, inactive against penicillin-resistant strains of staphylococci, and not highly bound to serum protein. Chemically, it is alpha-carboxybenzylpenicillin.

Carbenicillin appears to be virtually nontoxic and has no local irritant effects;[26] reports of changes in hepatic, renal, or hemopoietic function have not yet appeared, although the potential to cause hypersensitivity reactions such as drug fever and eosinophilia has been reported by some investigators. Carbenicillin appears to be well tolerated when administered intramuscularly or intravenously. However, it is not absorbed following oral administration. It passes with difficulty into the cerebrospinal fluid.

Since carbenicillin has a low toxicity effect, it is possible to prescribe large doses for prolonged time periods. However, investigators indicate that superinfection is enhanced following carbenicillin therapy.[27] In part, this may be caused by the effects of either a complex therapeutic regimen, steroids, or by immunosuppressive and cytotoxic agents. Other investigators suggest that strains of *Pseudomonas pyocyanea* emerging with an increase in resistance to carbenicillin may be overcome by administering carbenicillin and gentamicin as a synergistic combination.[28]

Studies on the intraocular penetration of carbenicillin in human beings following subconjunctival injection are under investigation.

Other drugs

The cephalosporins

The cephalosporins are semisynthetic antimicrobial agents derived from a *Cephalosporium* species of fungus. The molecular structure of the nucleus of these chemotherapeutic agents shows a similarity to the penicillins in containing a beta-lactam ring. Cephalosporins are bactericidal, and their mechanism of antibacterial activity is identical to the penicillins, resulting in inhibition of bacterial cell wall synthesis. Cephalosporin derivatives have been introduced clinically because they possess a broader antibacterial range than most penicillins (being active against some gram-negative organisms) and because they possess a relative resistance to penicillinase.

Cephalothin

Cephalothin (Keflin), a derivative of cephalosporin C, is highly active in vitro against the commonly encountered gram-positive bacteria, including penicillinase-producing staphylococci, and is also active against many gram-negative bacilli. For broad-spectrum therapy of infections before identification of the etiologic agent, cephalothin should be very useful and, on occasion, preferable to chloramphenicol and ampicillin. Individuals with known sensitivity to penicillin usually have tolerated cephalothin without untoward effects. The availability of such an agent represents an important advance in antibiotic therapy.

Cephalothin is generally well tolerated, but with higher doses or more frequent administration, a marked degree of pain occurs with intramuscular injection. Irritation of veins with intravenous administrations has also occurred, but these problems have rarely led to the need to discontinue therapy with cephalothin. Rashes, urticaria, and eosinophilia have been reported by a number of investigators, but the incidence is below 50%. Evidence of cross-sensitivity between cephalothin (Keflin) and penicillin is beginning to appear.

Studies of cephalothin levels in human secondary aqueous humor following intravenous injection and in rabbit primary aqueous humor after intramuscular injection show that this antibiotic reaches ocular levels that may be therapeutically effective against susceptible pathogens. No untoward reaction other than an occasional bitter taste was noted after the rapid, intravenous injection.[29, 30]

Studies of the intraocular penetration of cephalothin in human beings following subconjunctival injection are under investigation.

Cephaloridine

Therapeutically, cephaloridine appears to offer several advantages over cephalothin, although in vitro both antibiotics demonstrate a similar degree of activity against susceptible gram-positive and gram-negative organisms. These antibiotics must be given parenterally, but cephaloridine is more soluble and less painful when injected intramuscularly. Serum levels of cephaloridine are higher and more prolonged than those of cephalothin. In addition, cephalothin is 40% protein bound whereas no significant protein binding of cephaloridine has been demonstrated (Kunim and Atuk, 1966[30a]). The limitation of cephaloridine is that large doses (over 4 gm. per day) should not be given because of its potential for nephrotoxicity.

Preliminary studies of ocular penetration of cephaloridine and cephalothin in rabbits demonstrated significant levels in the aqueous humor, although little was found in the vitreous humor.[31]

Riley, Boyle, and Leopold[32] demonstrated that intramuscularly administered cephaloridine reaches the aqueous humor of noninflamed human eyes in levels that may be therapeutically effective. One gram of cephaloridine administered every 6 hours appears sufficient to maintain effective aqueous humor levels.

Records[33] confirmed the penetration studies of earlier workers on the experimental animal. In addition, he noted significant concentrations to be present in primary aqueous humor from 30 minutes to 2 hours following a single injection of 1 gm. intravenously.

High and prolonged antibiotic concentrations were detected in secondary aqueous humor after doses of the same size were administered similarly.

Patients hypersensitive to the penicillins and to whom a parenteral medication is necessary have been treated with the cephalosporin derivatives, cephaloridine or cephalothin, and it has been shown that some patients can show a cross-sensitivity between the cephalosporins. Therefore, a close observation of patients undergoing such therapy should be maintained, particularly where an allergic history exists.

Studies of the intraocular penetration of cephaloridine in human beings following subconjunctival injection are under investigation.

Cephalexin

Cephalexin is a new orally absorbed semisynthetic antibiotic derivative of cephalosporin. Like the other congeners of cephalosporanic acid, it interferes with bacterial cell wall synthesis and is also resistant to the action of penicillinase. Cephalexin has a broad spectrum of antimicrobial activity and a minimal serum protein binding potential; and in contrast to cephalothin and cephaloridine, it is well absorbed, and therapeutic levels are achieved in human serum following oral administration. Studies on ocular penetration in the rabbit and in man indicate that detectable levels of cephalexin appear in the aqueous humor of the noninflamed eye following oral administration.[34, 35]

In man cephalexin is rapidly absorbed from the gastrointestinal tract, and investigators have infrequently reported that it causes a minimal amount of nausea, vomiting, abdominal cramps, diarrhea, eosinophilia, rash, elevation of serum hepatic enzymes, and a positive reaction to Coomb's test. Reports of nephrotoxicity have not appeared to date. Patients allergic to penicillin have received cephalexin uneventfully, although the question of cross-allergenicity between the cephalosporins and the penicillins is still being investigated. Investigators have shown that infections caused by penicillin-sensitive and penicillin-resistant staphylococci, pneumococci, streptococci, *Klebsiella* species, *Escherichia coli,* and *Proteus mirabilis* were effectively treated with cephalexin without adverse reaction or significant toxicity.[36] Therefore, cephalexin, because of its ocular level of penetration in man following oral administration, its reported lack of nephrotoxicity, its broad spectrum of antimicrobial activity, and its nonallergic potential, augurs well for its inclusion as a therapeutic agent against susceptible pathogens in ocular infection.

Lincomycin

Lincomycin (Lincocin) is effective against most gram-positive bacteria, including staphylococci, streptococci, and pneumococci. Penicillin-resistant strains of staphylococci are often susceptible. Resistant organisms have been encountered, but usually after prolonged therapy. Lincomycin may be either bacteriocidal or bacteriostatic. This is usually determined by the concentration of the antibiotic and the susceptibility of the organism.

Ocular penetration studies have shown that theoretically adequate concentrations of lincomycin can be obtained in the noninflamed human eye when the drug is administered parenterally or subconjunctivally.[37, 38] Adverse reactions seemed limited to a rather marked chemosis that appeared within a few minutes of injection and that subsided considerably after a few hours time following subconjunctival administration. Patients complained of little or no pain when the antibiotic was administered, and no adverse systemic effects were noted in any of the patients so studied.

Lincomycin may be given orally, subconjunctivally, intramuscularly, and intravenously, as well as locally. The aqueous humor levels obtained are similar to that shown for other leading antibiotics, and the drug could be useful when administered to patients with ocular infections caused by gram-positive pathogens susceptible to lincomycin.

No serious side effects have been encountered to date. Hypersensitivity occurs infrequently, and the drug may be used in patients with known sensitivity to penicillin.

Polymyxin B and colistin

Ocular infections caused by gram-negative bacilli—in particular, *Pseudomonas* infections—are of considerable concern to the ophthalmologist. Polymyxin B has been most useful in the *Pseudomonas* infections. Colistin (Coly-Mycin) was introduced in 1961, and its ocular penetration and tolerance was reported in 1962. Colistin was recognized to resemble polymyxin pharmacologically and chemically to a remarkable extent. Further ocular penetration and tolerance studies at The Wills Eye Hospital demonstrated little difference in the two derivatives in methane sulfonate or sulfate forms.

Methane sulfonate preparations of each compound were less irritating than the sulfate, but the sulfate form of each has been shown to be a trifle more effective than the methane sulfonate in both bacteriostatic and bacteriocidal activity against *Pseudomonas.* Polymyxin B sulfate was a little more effective than either the sulfate or the methane sulfonate of colistin.

Gentamicin

Gentamicin (Garamycin) is a relatively new antibiotic that is active against a wide variety of gram-negative and gram-positive bacteria. It is unique as an antibiotic, for it is clinically active against *Pseudomonas* and *Proteus,* as well as *Staphylococcus* species. Gentamicin has been shown to be active against bacteria resistant to other antibiotics, such as neomycin and kanamycin.

The drug is stable in aqueous solution. It may be given intramuscularly or locally. It has been approved by the Food and Drug Administration. Phototoxicity has been reported, and impaired renal function may produce high blood levels in patients taking this drug. The risk of vestibular damage is greater in patients who may have impaired renal function. Gentamicin may be useful to ophthalmology as another mechanism for controlling *Pseudomonas* infections as well as other severe gram-negative infections of the corneal or intraocular structures.

Studies on ocular penetration following subconjunctival injection in the rabbit show that the antibiotic was well tolerated and produced adequate inhibitory levels in primary and secondary aqueous humor of the noninflamed eye.[39, 40] In addition, experimental data of ocular tissue absorption of gentamicin suggest that a sub-Tenon's injection would give at least the minimum inhibitory concentration for susceptible bacteria in most of the ocular tissues.[41] Studies following subconjunctival injection show that in man noninflamed eye levels that would be effective against susceptible pathogens were achieved in the aqueous humor.[42] Investigators in clinical studies confirm the effectiveness of gentamicin when administered topically in cases of human conjunctivitis in which the antibiotic was well tolerated.[43, 44, 45]

It has been suggested that the emergence of resistant strains may be prevented by the antimalarial quinacrine (Atabrine) hydrochloride, acting in combination with various antibiotics and sulfonamides. Quinacrine may prevent the emergence of bacterial strains resistant to streptomycin, penicillin, chloramphenicol, erythromycin, tetracycline, and novobiocin. It does not appear to be as effective once the bacterial strains have developed resistance. It seems only to prevent the resistance-inducing action of antibiotics on normal bacteria. This property of quinacrine has not been explored in ophthalmology.

In the field of ocular syphilis, recovery of treponemal organisms in the aqueous humor and the use of FTA absorption tests have led to the possibility that there are cases of ocular syphilis responsible for uveal disease that may not be recognized in any other fashion. It is not clear that all of these that have been diagnosed in this fashion are truly cases of active syphilitic infection. Some of the FTA absorption tests have given equivocal results in a few patients. There is always the possibility that nonpathogenic treponemes, such as *T. microdentium*, might on occasion penetrate the eye, since it is known that transient bacteremia may result from organisms that normally inhabit the mouth.

Treatment of presumed ocular syphilis with ampicillin and probenecid (Benemid) has not been entirely successful. Attempts have been made to treat such cases with erythromycin with some success. Recently, parenterally administered cephaloridine has been used in the therapy of patients with early syphilis, with sufficient benefit to warrant further study.[46]

MANAGEMENT OF INTRAOCULAR INFECTION

Prophylactic antibiotics for intraocular surgery

There have been a number of reports demonstrating the value of prophylactic subconjunctival antibiotics in cataract surgery. The first report of this type was made by Pearlman in 1956. Cassady[47] recently reported a series of 1,212 cataract operations performed over the past decade without a single postoperative infection. Penicillin was injected under the inferior bulbar conjunctiva at the end operation in all cases. This included 52 patients who reported penicillin sensitivity; only 11.5% of the latter had an abnormal reaction that did not damage the eye in any instance. In the most recent administration gentamicin has been used in patients who have any history of penicillin sensitivity.

In the last twenty-nine operations colistin was combined with penicillin. It is interesting that although bacterial endophthalmitis could occur with a resistant organism despite prophylactic subconjunctival antibiotics, no cases occurred in a total of 4,438 cataract operations that received various antibiotics. This seems to justify routine use of subconjunctival antibiotics at the end of every cataract extraction. Hughes commented on this in the *Year Book of Ophthalmology*, 1969, and stated that in his own experience for over 20 years the value of prophylactic use of antibiotics after cataract extraction has been demonstrated. The use of antibiotics subconjunctivally does not imply that other antiinfectious measures should be neglected. Obviously, one must adopt the best possible aseptic conditions at the time of surgery.

Chalkley and Shoch[48] studied 852 patients who underwent uncomplicated cataract extraction at Passavant Memorial Hospital in Chicago; 571 received an injection of antibiotics into the subconjunctival space. None of these patients received any systemic or topical antibiotics. All of the patients were carefully prepared with surgical scrubs, and the cul-de-sacs were irrigated with physiologic saline. The study patients received an injection of 0.4 ml. of a solution containing 40,000 units of aqueous penicillin and 40 ml. of streptomycin. If penicillin sensitivity was suspected, 40 ml. of chloramphenicol was substituted. The eye was covered with a 10% sodium sulfacetamide ointment and was bandaged at the close of surgery. During the postoperative period, the same antibiotics were applied topically to the eye on each day for 2 to 3 weeks after surgery. No patient had any adverse reaction to the subconjunctival antibiotic.

Two hundred eighty-one control patients were treated similarly, but they did not receive subconjunctival antibiotics at the time of surgery. Endophthalmitis developed in two of the patients treated with antibiotics for an incidence of 0.35%. In both, the onset was delayed, and the infections ran an insidious course. *Proteus* was obtained in one case and no organism in the other. Phthisis bulbi developed in both cases. Endophthalmitis developed in two of the patients who received no antibiotics, an incidence of 0.71%. These infections developed on the first and third postoperative days, respectively. *Staphylococcus aureus* was obtained in one case and no organism in the other. One eye had to be enucleated 2 months after operation, and in the other retinal detachment surgery was performed 3 months after surgery. Both of these studies demonstrate favorable statistics for the use of subconjunctival antibiotics, but also point out that such a technique does not eliminate postoperative endophthalmitis, and it is no substitute for meticulous aseptic technique.

The management of intraocular infection requires prompt therapy. Cultures should be taken wherever possible as a guide in the selection of the proper antiinfectious therapy. However, this is not always possible, particularly in dealing with intraocular inflammations. The delicacy of the ocular tissues and the great difficulty they have in regaining functional integrity after once being damaged by a severe infection make antibacterial therapy of very little value unless it is instituted very early. One must assume that the intraocular infection is caused by the organisms usually incriminated, where cultures cannot be obtained. This would include staphylococci, streptococci, pneumococci, *Escherichia coli, Pseudomonas aeruginosa,* and *Proteus* species. Staphylococci may be of the penicillinase-producing type, and one therefore has to employ a drug that will destroy both gram-positive and gram-negative organisms.

There are certain conditions that will allow one to combine drugs. In such cases in which bacteriologic control is unavailable, one is justified in using a combination therapy that will attack a wide range of possible responsible organisms. It is possible that the infection may be caused by more than one organism, gram-positive as well as gram-negative agents, and therefore a combined therapy may be a necessity. Sometimes when an organism is not very susceptible to one agent, it may respond to two, each of which attacks a different phase of the metabolism of the organism.

To ensure therapeutic drug levels within the eye, subconjunctival as well as systemic therapy should be given. The subconjunctival route can be used for agents that when given systemically would be quite toxic, particularly when the dosage required to penetrate into the ocular tissues and fluid may need to be large, therefore endangering the vulnerable structures in the general system to a greater extent.

Recent antibiotic side effects

There is some evidence that certain antibiotics may induce a form of myasthenia. Studies on animals suggest that the combined use of kanamycin and colistin (Coly-Mycin) may produce a deficiency in the production of acetylcholine.

Some patients develop a positive reaction to Coombs' test when taking cephaloridine.

Resistant staphylococci

Although there are available at the present time a number of potentially excellent agents for the treatment of staphylococcal infection, we may not relax. A few years ago, it was evident that the *Staphylococcus* species had developed strains resistant to penicillin G, chloramphenicol, erythromycin, and tetracycline. Then the new semisynthetic penicillins were introduced, led by methicillin. This was the first penicillinase-resistant semisynthetic penicillin. It was followed rapidly by oxacillin, nafcillin and cloxacillin. Also, other agents were introduced and found to be effective against the resistant *Staphylococcus*. Among these were cephalothin, cephaloridine, linocomycin, and cephalexin.

Consequently, there was quite a strong force available with which to combat the resistant organism. Shortly after the introduction of methicillin, strains of staphylococci were encountered that were resistant to the drug. As the years have passed, it has become apparent that methicillin-resistant staphylococci were often not suppressed by other antimicrobial agents. These have been found all over the world and have been noted to emerge, spread, and persist in hospitals. Infections caused by them have been traced to sick and to healthy carriers. These strains were present before methicillin was introduced, but they do seem to develop more frequently in those hospitals in which the drug has been used extensively as compared with those in which it has been used less frequently.[31]

These organisms resistant to methicillin appear to be insensitive to penicillin G, streptomycin, erythromycin, kanamycin, chloramphenicol, and tetracycline. Some are insensitive to cephalothin and lincomycin.

In view of these observations, when the responsible organism cannot be determined, it may prove unwise to use as a cover either methicillin or a combination of methicillin with penicillin G or oxacillin or cloxacillin.

Bulger[24] suggested using the combination of kanamycin and cephalothin until in vitro testing results become available. However, this is infrequently possible in intraocular infections.

For ophthalmologic purposes, it seems preferable to use vancomycin. This compound has a high degree of anti-*Staphylococcus* efficiency and so far a total absence of demonstrated resistance. This may be because of its limited use to date. If it is frequently used in widespread fashion, it may lose this superiority and become another antibiotic to which the *Staphylococcus* develops resistance. The limited use of vancomycin is probably because of its toxicity. It can produce loss of hearing, renal damage, a shocklike state, and severe allergic—even anaphylactic—reactions. These are rare complications and should not deter ophthalmic surgeons from the judicious use of vancomycin. Nevertheless, it is apparent that the *Staphylococcus* problem remains.

If no improvement in intraocular infections is noted in 24 hours, other antibiotics must be selected. At this time adrenocorticotropic hormone (ACTH) or corticosteroid therapy, which has been withheld, may be started. Usually ACTH or corticosteroid therapy is withheld until after the first 24 hours of antibacterial therapy because these anti-inflammatory agents may mask the influence of the antibiotic. They certainly will not be helpful unless the proper antibiotic to control the specific etiologic factor can be found. In severe cases, one can try direct injection of the antibiotic into the chambers of the eye.

Use of steroids

In dealing with intraocular infection, it is difficult to decide whether or not to use steroids. The most to be gained would be the reduction of the inflammatory reaction. Useful vision has been lost in spite of halting an infectious process because of the extensive inflammatory damage resulting from the infection. Steroids have been recommended to reduce this damage to allow time for specific medication to become effective.

Experimental studies have demonstrated that steroids usually do not interfere with the effectiveness of a specific antibiotic administered in dosage adequate to overcome an infection caused by a sensitive organism.[49] However, there is no proof that the eventual result is superior when steroids are used in combination with an effective antibiotic rather than when the antibiotic is used alone.

Recently, Freeman and Gay[10] questioned the value of steroids in conjunction with antibiotics for the management of intraocular infections after cataract surgery.

In 37 infected eyes, 15 were treated with antibiotics alone. Twelve of these had resultant visual acuity of 20/100 or better. Of 22 eyes treated with antibiotics and steroids, 11 had resultant acuities exceeding 20/100. Two of the 15 treated with antibiotics alone were lost, and two of the 22 treated with antibiotics and steroids were lost. These results may not be statistically significant but certainly do not demonstrate a decided superiority for either approach. There are many variables that are difficult to evaluate. These statistics are remarkable in that only 4 eyes of the 37 analyzed were totally lost, just a trifle over 10%. The organism in one of these was *Pseudomonas,* in another *Proteus,* and in one hemolytic *Staphylococcus.* In 5 recently reported outbreaks, 25 eyes were lost after 40 infections (63%), all caused by *Pseudomonas.* In the overwhelming majority, only antibiotics had been employed.

In another study, 22 infections were analyzed. Twelve of the eyes revealed *Staphylococcus aureus,* 4 *Pseudomonas aeruginosa,* 3 *Pneumococcus,* 2 *Escherichia coli,* 1 *Streptococcus,* and 1 *Proteus.* Some of the eyes produced more than one pathogen. Seventeen of these eyes were lost. Three of the 5 saved had *Staphylococcus aureus,* one had *Proteus,* and the other cultured *Pseudomonas* and *Escherichia coli.*

In this second series of culture infections, the salvage rate was approximately 23% (5/22), 77% being lost.

In other words, where *Pseudomonas* was definitely the known offending organism, only 15 out of 40 were salvaged in one series. Where the organisms were predominantly *Staphylococcus,* 31 of 37 were shown to retain some visual function. These observations stress the importance of the responsible organism in determining the outcome. It may be that these eyes treated with steroids and antibiotics have done remarkably well. The resistance of the host, the size of the inoculum, and the virulence of the infecting agent are all difficult criteria to control in any clinical study.

The virulence and drug resistance of the organisms in those managed with combined treatment may have been more pronounced than in those treated with antibiotics alone.

There are a number of eyes in the Freeman-Gay[10] series in which the steroids were not used in the first 24 hours of therapy. This suggests that the initially selected antibiotic regimen was not successful, and steroids may have been introduced to retard the inflammatory onslaught while other antibiotics were introduced specifically to stop the advancing infection.

The use of steroids in the management of intraocular infections remains an undecided clinical problem. Perhaps a useful guide here is to use the hormonal agents only if the initially selected antibiotics fail to show a favorable effect on the ocular involvement, and perhaps late in the course to further reduce inflammatory damage in eyes responding to antibiotic therapy. Whenever steroids are used, the eye must be monitored meticulously.

Relative cost of medication

In ocular infections cost is not the most important factor, but one should not be unaware of this in our present society. Table 13-6 lists

Table 13-6. Comparative cost of antibiotics*

Drug	*Average daily dose*	*Dose form*	*Average daily cost*
Ampicillin (Polycillin)	6 gm.	Oral	$ 2.40
	4 gm.	I.M., I.V.	4.00
Carbenicillin (Pyopen)	30 gm.	I.M.	123.37
Cephalothin (Keflin)	6 gm.	I.M., I.V.	21.30
Cephaloridine (Kefloridin)	4 gm.	I.M.	21.20
	25 mg.	Subconjunctival	0.13
Cephalexin (Keflex)	4 gm.	Oral	12.80
Chloramphenicol (Chloromycetin)	6 gm.	Oral	4.80
	8 gm.	I.V.	7.60
Colistin (Coly-Mycin)	150 mg.	I.M.	7.25
Erythromycin (Erythrocin)	4 gm.	Oral	3.60
Gentamicin (Garamycin)	210 mg. (1 mg./kg.)	I.M.	1.48
Lincomycin (Lincocin)	2.8 gm.	I.M.	14.00
	50 mg.	Subconjunctival	0.25
Methicillin (Staphcillin)	8 gm.	I.M., I.V.	26.00
Oxacillin (Prostaphlin)	8 gm.	Oral	8.00
Penicillin	1.2 million units	I.M.	1.00
	10 million units	I.V.	2.00
Tetracycline	3 gm.	Oral	1.80
	2 gm.	I.V.	4.80
Streptomycin	2 gm.	I.M.	2.00

*Pharmacy Department, The Mount Sinai Hospital, New York, April 1971.

the relative cost for daily therapy in one major hospital. The use of the more expensive antibiotics should be restricted to those situations in which there is a clear medical indication.

ANTIFUNGAL AGENTS

Many chemotherapeutic agents have been developed during the past decade for the management of superficial and deep fungus infection. Some are antibiotics, such as amphotericin B, nystatin, and griseofulvin (Fulvicin). Others are chemical compounds that have selective specific action against certain individual fungi but are not antibiotics, such as tolnaftate (Tinactin) and hydroxystilbamidine isethionate.

In previous decades superficial mycotic infections were treated with keratolytic agents, such as benzoic acid, salicylic acid, undecylenic and propionic acid. These have been relatively ineffective compounds.

In recent years the incidence of opportunistic infections caused by true fungi and higher bacteria has increased strikingly. This may be related to the increased use of antimicrobials and glucocorticosteroids, the growing reservoir of patients with chronic debilitating disease, the growing use of immunosuppressive drugs as tissue transplantation increases, the implantation of foreign materials such as silicone and plastics, and to bolder surgery.

The organisms commonly occurring in these situations include *Nocardia asteroides, Cryptococcus neoformans,* and species of *Mucor, Aspergillus,* and *Monilia (Candida).* Over half the patients who develop nocardiosis either have severe underlying diseases, such as leukemia, lymphoma, carcinoma, or alveolar proteinosis, or they have received large doses of adrenal steroid hormones.

Mucormycosis usually complicates uncontrolled diabetes, burns, and neoplastic and inflammatory diseases. It is seen also where there has been malnutrition and serious gastrointestinal disorders.

Similarly, torulosis is said to occur more frequently in diabetics, in patients receiving steroids, and in those with hypogammaglobulinemia. However, many patients who have this disorder have no obvious underlying disease.

Aspergilli are common contaminants, and isolations must be carefully evaluated and correlated to clinical situations before being discarded as contaminants. Usually aspergillosis is seen where there has been a severe underlying illness. Patients with chronic asthma and bronchitis, as well as those treated with antibiotics and steroids and those with bronchiectasis, seem to have a penchant for the condition.

Candidiasis, histoplasmosis, or coccidioidomycosis may occur as opportunistic infection. We rarely see secondary infections or direct infections of the eye by the *Mycobacterium tuberculosis.* There appears to be a rising incidence of corneal and, occasionally, intraocular infections caused by mycobacteria of atypical varieties. Attention was called to these organisms as a potential for human disease many years ago.[50] Four groups have been defined.

Group I includes photochromogens representing a relatively homogeneous group termed "mycobacteria kansasii." These produce pulmonary disease.

Group II consists of scotochromogens, which are infrequent human pathogens that can produce pulmonary or lymph node disease.

Group III is made up of the nonchromogens, known also as the Battey group. These are prominent human pathogens in certain geographic areas, such as southeastern United States and western Australia. They produce both pulmonary and disseminate disease.

Group IV, the so-called rapid-growing acid-fast bacilli, contains diverse strains. One of these strains, *Mycobacterium fortuitum,* is an occasional pulmonary pathogen for man. At The Mount Sinai Hospital[51] and in the Armed Forces Institute of Pathology, this has been encountered as a definite cause of corneal and intraocular infection. All of these unclassified mycobacteria are more resistant to chemotherapy than is *Myco-*

Table 13-7. Intravenous drug incompatibility*

Drugs (antibiotics)	*Incompatible with*
Ampicillin sodium (Penbritin)	Manufacturer recommends addition of no other solution
Amphotericin B (Fungizone)	Potassium penicillin G, tetracyclines (should be administered alone)
Cephalothin (Keflin)	Calcium chloride or gluconate, erythromycin lactobionate, polymyxin B, tetracyclines (Manufacturer recommends that drug be administered alone)
Chloramphenicol sodium succinate (Chloromycetin)	B-complex vitamins, hydrocortisone, erythromycin, polymyxin B, prochlorperazine, tetracyclines, vancomycin
Methicillin (Staphcillin)	Kanamycin sulfate, metaraminol, tetracyclines, vancomycin
Penicillin G potassium	Amphotericin B, heparin sodium, metaraminol, phenylephrine, tetracyclines, vancomycin
Polymyxin B	Cephalothin, chloramphenicol, heparin, tetracyclines
Tetracyclines	Amphotericin B, cephalothin, chloramphenicol, heparin, hydrocortisone, methicillin, potassium penicillin G, polymyxin B
Vancomycin (Vancocin)	Chloramphenicol, heparin, hydrocortisone, methicillin, potassuim penicillin G, sulfisoxazole diethanolamine

*Adapted from Formulary Facts, The Mount Sinai Hospital, issue 18, September 1967.

therapy. Smears may be stained by the Gram method or in 10% potassium hydroxide mounts, or with periodic acid–Schiff reaction stain.

INTRAVENOUS DRUG INCOMPATIBILITY

The use of the intravenous method of administration of drugs has increased in recent years, and with this increase, a tendency to mix drugs has developed. It is the physician who prescribes medication, so he must be aware of the common incompatibilities he may encounter.

A physically visible incompatibility does not necessarily indicate a therapeutic inactivation, nor does the absence of a visible physical sign of incompatibility indicate that a therapeutic incompatibility has not occurred.

It is recommended that solutions showing evidence of a physical incompatibility be discarded and drugs be administered singularly.

Table 13-7 lists a few common incompatibilities that may develop in the mixing of solutions for intravenous drip administration.

ANTIPROTOZOAL DRUGS

Protozoal organisms may give rise to ocular disease. Some of these protozoa may be ingested such as *Entamoeba histolytica* or *Giardia lamblia.* Both of these agents have been incriminated rightly or wrongly in uveal disease. Most of the pathogenic protozoa, however, are conveyed to the human host by an insect or vector in which the pathogen passes a part of its life cycle; for example, the *Toxoplasma* may be carried by *Toxocara canis.*

One method of ridding a community of vector-borne disease is to attack the vector. Many insecticides have been developed for this purpose.

Resistance to protozoal infection can develop, and hereditary forms of protozoal resistance have been described. Many of the agents used in the fight against protozoal diseases are of importance to ophthalmology. They have been used for treatment of ocular diseases. Several of these agents have toxic effects for ocular structures (Table 13-8).

Table 13-8. Protozoal infection

Organism	*Disease*	*Drug of choice*	*Maximal daily adult dose*
Toxoplasma	Uveitis	Pyrimethamine (Daraprim)	0.35 to 1.50 mg./kg.
		Sulfonamides	4 gm.
Entamoeba histolytica	Dysentery	Emetine hydrochloride	1 mg./kg.
	Chorioretinitis(?)	Diiodohydroxyquinoline	2.5 gm.
		Chloroquine diphosphate	750 mg.
Giardia lamblia	Uveitis(?)	Meparacrine hydrochloride	1 mg./kg.
Plasmodium	Malaria	Prophylaxis	
		Amodiaquine hydrochloride (Camoquin)	300 mg. same day each week
		Chloroquine diphosphate	500 mg. same day each week
		Treatment	
		Amodiaquine hydrochloride (Camoquin)	600 mg.
		Chloroquine diphosphate	900 mg.
Leishmania donovani	Lid infections	Sodium stibogluconate	600 mg.
	Retinal hemorrhage	Pentamidine	4 mg./kg.
	Iridocyclitis		
Trypanosoma	Keratitis	Prophylaxis	
	Iridocyclitis	Pentamidine	3 mg./kg.
	Sleeping sickness	Early treatment	
		Suramin sodium	1 gm.
		Late treatment	90 mg.
		Melarsoprol	

SUMMARY

Antibiotic and chemotherapeutic agents employed for ophthalmic therapy can produce local and systemic toxicity. The type and frequency of these side effects and complications can depend on the agents, the dosage and duration of therapy, and the individual susceptibility. The dosage schedule should be selected on the basis of penetration. Agent selection usually must be made without bacteriologic identification of the organism. The routes of administration are recommended on the basis of optimal penetration, minimal toxicity, patient tolerance, and clinical experience.

REFERENCES

1. Thoburn, R., Fekety, F. R., Jr., and others: Infections acquired by hospitalized patients, Arch. Intern. Med. **121**:1, 1968.
2. Allen, H. F., and Mangiaracine, A. B.: Bacterial endophthalmitis after cataract extraction, Arch. Ophthal. **72**:454, 1964.
3. Ayliffe, G. A. J., Barry, D. R., and others: Postoperative infection with Pseudomonas aeruginosa in an eye hospital, Lancet **1**:113, 1966.
4. Allen, H. F.: Aseptic techniques in ophthalmology, Trans. Amer. Acad. Ophthal. Otolaryng. **57**:377, 1959.
5. Crompton, D. P.: Personal observations in the preventing of sepsis. In Theodore, F. A., editor: Complications after cataract extraction, Boston, 1964, Little, Brown & Co. p. 509.
6. Blowers, R.: Content of infection in ophthalmic surgery, Proc. Roy. Soc. Med. **60**:351, 1967.
7. Lowbury, E. J. L.: Control of infection in ophthalmic surgery, Proc. Roy. Soc. Med. **60**:349, 1967.
8. Lowbury, E. J. L., Lilly, H. A., and Bull, J. P.: Methods for disinfection of hands and operation sites, Brit. Med. J. **5408**:531, 1964.
9. Nolan, J.: Evaluation of conjunctival and nasal bacterial cultures before intraocular operations, Brit. J. Ophthal. **51**:483, 1967.
10. Freeman, M. I., and Gay, A. J.: Systemic steroid therapy in postcataract endophthalmitis. In Becker, E. B., and Drews, R. C., editors: Current concepts in ophthalmology, St. Louis, 1967, The C. V. Mosby Co.
11. Sarconi, I.: Drug allergies, Proc. Roy. Soc. Med. **61**:891, 1968.
12. DeWeck, A. L.: Penicillin allergy: its detection by an improved haemagglutination technique, Nature **202**:975, 1964.
13. Tuft, L., Gregory, D. C., and Gregory, J.: Evaluation of skin testing methods employed in diagnosis of penicillin allergy, Amer. J. Med. Sci. **230**:370, 1955.
14. Parker, C. W., DeWeck, A. L., and others: The preparation and some properties of penicillinic acid derivatives relevant to penicillin hypersensitivity, J. Exp. Med. **115**:803, 1962.
15. Levine, B. B., and Price, V. H.: Studies on the immunological mechanisms of penicillin allergy. II. Antigenic specificities of allergic wheal-and-flare skin responses in patients with histories of penicillin allergy, Immunology **7**:542, 1964.
16. Siegel, B. B., and Levine, B. B.: Antigenic specificities of skin-sensitizing antibodies in sera from patients with immediate systemic allergic reactions to penicillin, J. Allerg. **35**:488, 1964.
17. Shelley, W. B.: Indirect basophil degranulation test for allergy to penicillin and other drugs, J. A. M. A. **184**:171, 1963.
18. Katz, H. I., Gill, K. A., and others: Indirect basophil degranulation test in penicillin allergy, J. A. M. A. **188**:351, 1964.

19. Shelley, W. B., and Comaish, J. S.: New test for penicillin allergy: fluorometric assay of histamine release, J. A. M. A. **192**:36, 1965.
20. Halpern, B., and Amache, H.: Diagnosis of drug allergy in vitro with the lymphocyte transformation test, J. Allerg. **40**:168, 1967.
21. Kunin, C. M.: Effects of antibiotics on gastrointestinal tract, Clin. Pharmacol. Ther. **8**:495, 1967.
22. Brauninger, G. E., and Remington, I. L.: Nephropathy associated with methicillin therapy, J. A. M. A. **203**:103, 1968.
23. Benner, S. J., and Morthland, V.: Methicillin-resistant Staphylococcus aureus, New Eng. J. Med. **277**:678, 1967.
24. Bulger, R. J.: Methicillin-resistant strain of Staphylococcus aureus, Ann. Intern. Med. **67**:8189, 1967.
25. Farrar, W. E., Jr., O'Dell, N. M., and Krause, J. M.: Use of penicillinase resistant penicillins to increase susceptibility of gram negative bacteria to antibiotics, Ann. Intern. Med. **67**:733, 1967.
26. Acred, P., Brown, D. M., and others: New semi-synthetic penicillin active against Pseudomonas pyocyanea, Nature **215**:25, 1967.
27. Marks, M. I., and Eickhoff, T. C.: Carbenicillin: a clinical and laboratory evaulation, Ann. Intern. Med. **72**:179, 1970.
28. Hoffman, T. A., and Bullock, W. E.: Carbenicillin therapy of Pseudomonas and other gram-negative bacillary infections, Ann. Intern. Med. **73**:165, 1970.
29. Records, R. E.: Intraocular penetration of cephalothin. II. Human studies, Amer. J. Ophthal. **66**:411, 1968.
30. Uwaydah, M. M., and Faris, B. M.: Penetration of cephalothin in the aqueous humor of the rabbit, Arch. Ophthal. **83**:349, 1970.
30a. Kunin, C. M., and Atuk, N.: Excretion of cephaloridine and cephalothin in patients with renal impairment, New Eng. J. Med. **274**:654, 1966.
31. Mizukawa, T., Azuma, I., and Kawaguchi, S.: Intraocular distribution of cephalothin and cephalorine, J. Antibiot. **18**:525, 1965.
32. Riley, F. C., Boyle, G. L., and Leopold, I. H.: Intraocular penetration of cephaloridine, in humans, Amer. J. Ophthal. **66**:1042, 1968.
33. Records, R. E.: Intraocular penetration of cephaloridine: observations in experimental animal and human eyes, Arch. Ophthal. **81**:331, 1969.
34. Gager, W. E., Elsas, F. J., and Lawton-Smith, J.: Ocular penetration of cephalexin in the rabbit, Brit. J. Ophthal. **53**:403, 1969.
35. Boyle, G. L., Hein, H. F., and Leopold, I. H.: Intraocular penetration of cephalexin in man, Amer. J. Ophthal. **69**:868, 1970.
36. Fass, R. J., Perkins, R. L., and Saslaw, S.: Cephalexin—a new oral cephalosporin: clinical evaluation in sixty-three patients, Amer. J. Med. Sci. **259**:187, 1970.
37. Becker, E. F.: The intraocular penetration of lincomycin, Amer. J. Ophthal. **67**:963, 1969.
38. Boyle, G. L., Lichtig, M. L., and Leopold, I. H.: Lincomycin levels in human ocular fluids and serum following subconjunctival injection, Amer. J. Ophthal. **71**:1303, 1971.
39. Furgiuele, F. P.: The ocular penetration and tolerance of gentamicin, Amer. J. Ophthal. **64**:421, 1967.
40. Litwalk, K. D., Pettit, T., and Lamar-Johnson, B.: Penetration of gentamicin, Arch. Ophthal. **82**:687, 1969.
41. Golden, B., and Coppel, S. P.: Ocular tissue absorption of gentamicin, Arch. Ophthal. **84**:792, 1970.
42. Furgiuele, F. P.: Penetration of gentamicin into the aqueous humor of human eyes, Amer. J. Ophthal. **69**:481, 1970.
43. Magnuson, R. H., and Suie, T.: Gentamicin sulfate in external eye infections, J. A. M. A. **199**:427, 1967.
44. Bras, J. F., and Coyle-Gilcrist, M. M.: Genticin in conjunctivitis and keratitis, Brit. J. Ophthal. **52**:560, 1968.

45. Magnuson, R. H., and Suie, T.: Clinical and bacteriologic evaluations of gentamicin ophthalmic preparations, Amer. J. Ophthal. **70**:734, 1970.
46. Glieksman, J. M., Short, D. H., and Knox, J.: Parenteral cephaloridine in treatment of patients with early syphilis, Arch. Intern. Med. **121**:342, 1968.
47. Cassady, J. R.: Prophylactic subconjunctival antibiotics following cataract extraction, Amer. J. Ophthal. **64**:1081, 1967.
48. Chalkley, T. H. F., and Shoch, D.: Evaluation of prophylactic subconjunctival antibiotic injection in cataract surgery, Amer. J. Ophthal. **64**:1084, 1969.
49. Leopold, I. H., and Maylath, F.: Intraocular penetration of cortisone and its effectiveness against experimental corneal burns, Amer. J. Ophthal. **35**:1125, 1952.
50. Timpe, A., and Runyon, E. H.: The relationship of atypical acid-fast bacteria to human diseases: preliminary report, J. Lab. Clin. Med. **44**:202, 1954.
51. Wunsh, S. F., Boyle, C. L., and others: Mycobacterium fortuitum infection of corneal graft, Arch. Ophthal. **82**:602, 1969.
52. Jenkins, D. E., and Wolinsky, E.: Mycobacterial diseases of the lung and bronchial tree. In Baum, G. L., editor: Textbook of pulmonary diseases, Boston, 1965, Little, Brown & Co., p. 256.
53. Phillips, S., and Larkin, J. C.: Atypical pulmonary tuberculosis caused by unclassified Mycobacterium, Ann. Intern. Med. **60**:401, 1964.
54. Robinson, H. M., Jr., and Rafkin, J.: Tolnaftate therapy of mycotic infections, J. Invest. Derm. **42**:185, 1964.
55. Giles, C. L., and Falls, H. F.: Amphotericin B therapy in the treatment of presumed Histoplasma chorioretinitis, Trans. Amer. Ophthal. Soc. **65**:136, 1967.
56. Newell, F. W.: Problems in use of anticancer agents in ophthalmology. In Leopold, I. H., editor: Ocular therapy: complications and management, vol. 1., St. Louis, 1966, The C. V. Mosby Co., p. 79.
57. Theodore, F. H., Littman, M. L., and Almeda, E.: Diagnosis and management of fungus endophthalmitis following cataract extraction, Arch. Ophthal. **66**:163, 1961.

Index

A

Abnormality, chemical, 2-3
Acetyl transferase, 97
Acetylation, 97
Acetylcholine, 30
Acetylsalicylic acid, 123
Achromycin; *see* Tetracycline
Acid; *see* specific acid
Acrisorcin, 145
Actase, 59
ACTH; *see* Adrenocorticotropic hormone
Action of dextran, mechanisms of, 58
Activity
  antiinflammatory and mineralocorticoid, of some corticosteroids, comparison of, 71
  glucocerebrosidase, 9-13
  sphingomyelinase, 14-15
Acuity, visual, 80, 87
Adenine arabinoside, 46-47
Adenosine diphosphate, 56
Adenosine triphosphate, 24
Administration
  drug, route of, 126
  topical mydriatic, average increase in pupillary diameter after, 101
ADP; *see* Adenosine diphosphate
Adrenocorticotropic hormone, 70, 74, 141
Adverse reactions, 30-33
Agents
  antifungal, 143-145
    systemic, 145-149
  available for management of fungal disease, 145-149
  hypoglycemic, 74
  immunosuppressive, in ophthalmology, 65-67
  lytic, and plasma expanders in ophthalmology, 55-63
  used to control infection, 126-129
Agglutination, platelet, 56
Akrinol; *see* Acrisorcin
ALA synthetase activity, 5
Albamycin sodium; *see* Novobiocin
Albinism, 20-22
Albumin, 57, 58
Allergy, 52
Allopurinol, 18
Amethopterin, 66
Amino acid metabolism, 19-24
Amino levulinic acid, 4, 5
6-Aminopenicillinic acid, 126
Aminophenyl, 121
Amniocentesis, diagnosis of heritable metabolic defects by, 26-28
Amodiaquine hydrochloride, 150
Amphotericin B, 37, 80, 84, 118, 125, 127, 143, 145, 146-147, 149
  use of, in chorioretinitis, 147-148
Ampicillin, 39, 50, 52, 80, 119, 124, 127, 129, 130, 132, 133, 137, 143, 149
Ancillin; *see* Diphencillin
Anesthetics, topical, 49
Antibiotic prophylaxis, 105-111
Antibiotic side effects, 140
Antibiotics, 36, 38-39, 48, 51, 54, 79, 80, 83, 138, 139, 141, 142, 144
  and chemotherapeutic substances, toxicity of, 118-119
  concentrated solutions of, for topical use, 51-53
  effectiveness study of, 105-111
  effects of, on gastrointestinal tract, 124-125
  problems in use of, in ophthalmology, 113-151
  prophylactic, for intraocular surgery, 138-139
  subconjunctival, 50-51
Antibiotic-steroid mixture, 54
Antibody
  gamma A, 44
  gamma G, 43
  gamma M, 43
Anticholinesterase, 34, 100
Anticoagulants, 55, 63

Antidiuretic hormone, 5
Antifungal agents, 143-145
  systemic, 145-149
Antiinflammatory and mineralocorticoid activity of some corticosteroids, comparison of, 71
Antimetabolites, 46, 65, 66, 67
Antimicrobial agents, toxicity of, 118
Antimicrobials, 84, 85, 113, 143
Antiprotozoal drugs, 149-150
6-APA; *see* 6-Aminopenicillinic acid
Applanation intraocular pressure; *see* Intraocular pressure, applanation
Arginine glutamate, 23
Aspergillus, 78, 144
Atabrine; *see* Quinacrine hydrochloride
Atropine, 34, 40, 54, 98, 99, 100, 102
  average increase in pupillary diameter after instillation of, 99
  increase in heart rate after instillation of, 99
Aureomycin; *see* Tetracycline
Axis, hypothalamic–pituitary–adrenal gland, 73, 74
Azathioprine, 66, 67, 147

B

Bacitracin, 39, 50, 52, 115, 118, 128
Bacteria, 81
Bacterial corneal ulcers, points in treatment of, 48-54; *see also* Points in treatment of bacterial corneal ulcers
Bacterial counts
  mean, 109
  postoperative, compared to preoperative, 109
Bacterial endophthalmitis, 39
Bacterial multiplication, 105-106
Barbiturates, 5, 97
Benemid; *see* Probenecid
Betamethasone, 71, 72, 90, 93, 98
Beta-N-acetyl galactosaminide, 16
Benzalkonium chloride, 115
Benzoic acid, 143
Benzo-penicillin, 121, 122
Benzyl penicillin, 132
Bishydroxycoumarin, 56, 57
Blastomyces, 146
Blepharoconjunctivitis, 31
Block
  in chain of chemical events within cell, 1
  pupillary, 31
Blood dyscrasias, 123-124
Brocillin; *see* Propicillin

C

Calcium gluconate, 75
Calcium lactate, 75
Camoquin; *see* Amodiaquine hydrochloride
Candida albicans, 78, 124, 144, 145, 146
Carbenicillin, 50, 52, 116, 127, 132-133, 143
Carbohydrates, 5-6
Cases, corticosteroid-treated, recurrent inflammation in, 86-87
Categories of inborn errors of metabolism, 3-4
Cell, block of chain of chemical events within, 1
Central stromal keratitis
  acute
    results of combined therapy in, 81
    results of combined therapy with keratoplasty in, 81
  infectious
    recurrent inflammation following combined therapy in, 81
    recurrent inflammation following penetrating keratoplasty in, 82
Cephalexin, 127, 135, 140, 143
Cephaloridine, 39, 50, 52, 116, 127, 128, 134-135, 137, 140, 143
Cephalosporin, 118, 132, 133, 135
Cephalosporium, 133, 148
Cephalothin, 39, 50, 52, 116, 127, 128, 132, 133-134, 135, 140, 143, 149
Ceramide trihexosidase, 7, 10, 17
Cerebral lipidoses, 7-8
Chemical abnormality, 2-3
Chemical events, block in chain of, within cell, 1
Chemipen; *see* Phenethicillin
Chemistry of Tay-Sachs disease, 16
Chemotherapeutic and antibiotic substances, toxicity of, 118-119
Children, toxicity of strong miotics in, 30-34
Chloramphenicol, 38, 39, 50, 51, 52, 79, 106, 107, 109, 110, 115, 118, 120, 124, 127, 128, 133, 137, 138, 140, 143, 149
Chlordiazepoxide, 5
Chlorhexide; *see* Chlorhexidine
Chlorhexidine, 115
Chlorobutanol, 115
Chlorocresol, 115
Chloromycetin; *see* Chloramphenicol
Chloroquine diphosphate, 150
Choice of penicillinase-resistant semisynthetic penicillin, 131-132
Cholesterol, 14
Chorioretinitis, use of amphotericin B in, 147-148

Classification of corneal disease, 78
Clostridium perfringens, 15
Clots, therapeutic measures for, 56-57
Cloxacillin, 118, 119, 129, 131, 140
Cocaine, 37, 40, 100, 101, 102, 103
Coccidioides, 146
Colistin, 39, 50, 52, 54, 118, 125, 127, 136, 138, 140, 143
Coly-Mycin; *see* Colistin
Committee on Thrombolytic Agents of National Heart Institute, 60
Comparison of antiinflammatory and mineralocorticoid activity of corticosteroids, 71
Complications and management of systemic corticosteroid therapy, 70-76
Concentrated solutions of antibiotics for topical use, 51-53
Conjunctival hyperemia, 31
Conjunctivitis, trachoma–inclusion, 78, 79, 80, 83
Coproporphyrin, 4
Corneal disease
  acute infectious peripheral
    recurrence of, 83
    results of combined therapy in, 83
  classification of, 78
  immunologic evaluation of, 79
  infectious, corticosteroids in, 77-87
  infiltrative, 80-84
  long-term patient follow-up on, 80
  patterns in therapy of, 79-80
  selection of patients with, 78-79
Corneal or peripheral ischemic disease, treatment of, 85-86
Corneal ulcers, smears of, 49
Correlation between recurrent inflammation and socioeconomic status, 82
Corticoid responsiveness, 97-98
Corticosteroid costs, 72
Corticosteroid responders, topical, use of medrysone in, 94
Corticosteroid testing, topical, intraocular pressure responses to, 40, 97
Corticosteroid therapy, systemic, management and complications of, 70-76
Corticosteroid-antimicrobial therapy in acute infectious corneal infiltrative diseases, 84-85
Corticosteroid-heparin therapy, combined, in infectious peripheral ischemic syndromes, 84
Corticosteroid-induced hypertension, 90
Corticosteroids, 36, 37, 38, 39-40, 43, 53, 54, 65, 66, 70, 71, 72, 73, 74, 75, 76, 77, 78, 79, 80, 82, 83, 84, 85, 86, 98, 141
Corticosteroids—cont'd
  comparison of antiinflammatory and mineralocorticoid activity of, 71
  daily therapeutic dosage of, 72
  diluted and new topical, intraocular pressure effects of, 90-95
  in infectious corneal disease, 77-87
  subconjunctival repository, 36, 37, 40
  topical
    elevation of applanation intraocular pressure after various dilutions of, 92
    various, applanation intraocular pressure of 24 patients after, 92
  trade names and tablet size of, 71
  various, mean applanation intraocular pressure after, 92, 93
Corticosteroid-treated cases, recurrent inflammation in, 86-87
Cortisol, 70, 71, 73
Cortisone, 39, 70, 76
Cost(s)
  corticosteroid, 72
  of medication, relative, 142-143
Coumarin, 97
Counts, bacterial; *see* Bacterial counts
Cremodiazine; *see* Sulfadiazine
Cryptococcus neoformans, 144, 146
Cul-de-sac disinfection, 115-116
Cultures, 49
Cyclitis, 40
Cyclophosphamide, 66, 67
Cycloserine, 118
Cysts, iris, 31
Cytochrome oxidase, 4

D

Daily observation, 53-54
Daily therapeutic dosage of corticosteroids, 72
Damage, eighth nerve, 125
Decadron; *see* Dexamethasone
Defects
  enzymatic, in sphingolipidoses, 8
  metabolic, heritable, diagnosis of, by amniocentesis, 26-28
Deficiency, pyridoxine, 6
Demerol; *see* Meperidine
Depletion, potassium, 75
Detachment, retinal, 31
Dexamethasone, 40, 54, 71, 72, 73, 74, 75, 79, 90, 91, 92, 93, 94, 95, 98
  topical elevation of applanation intraocular pressure after various dilutions of, 91
Dextran, 56, 57-59, 63
  mechanism of action of, 58

Dextran—cont'd
structural formula of, 57
Dextran 40, 58
Dextrose, 57
Diabetes, 74
Diagnosis of heritable metabolic defects by amniocentesis, 26-28
Diameter, pupillary; *see* Pupillary diameter, increase in
Difference in pressure and outflow facility after pilocarpine and epinephrine instillation, 103
Digitalis, 75
Dihydrostreptomycin, 125
Dihydroxyphenylalanine, 20
Diiodohydroxyquinoline, 150
Dilantin; *see* Sodium diphenylhydantoin
Diphenicillin, 129
Diphtheroids, 110
Disease
corneal; *see* Corneal disease
Fabry's, 17
fungal, agents available for management of, 145-149
Gaucher's, 8-13; *see also* Gaucher's disease
hepatic, 4
infectious corneal infiltrative, acute corticosteroid-antimicrobial therapy in, 84-85
liver, 125
Niemann-Pick, 13-15; *see also* Niemann-Pick disease
Refsum's, 6-7
reduction of substrate or precursors in, 7
Tay-Sachs, 15-17
Disinfection
cul-de-sac, 115-116
skin, 115
Dissolution, thrombus formation and, initiating mechanisms of, 55-56
Disturbance, gastrointestinal, 124-125
DNA, 2, 12, 13
Doraprim; *see* Pyrimethamine
Dosage, therapeutic daily, of corticosteroids, 72
Down's syndrome
drug sensitivity in, 98-100
hyperreactivity in, 33-34
Drug administration, route of, 126
Drug incompatibility, intravenous, 149
Drug responsiveness, racial or pigmentary influence on, 100-103
Drug sensitivity in Down's syndrome, 98-100
Drug usage and specific toxic effects, 119-126
Drugs
antiprotozoal, 149-150
newer, effects of, 130-138
and pharmacogenetics in ophthalmology, individual responsiveness to, 96-103
Dyscrasias, blood, 123-124

E

Echothiophate, 30, 31, 32, 33, 34, 40
systemic toxicity of, 32
Effectiveness study of antibiotics, 105-111
Effect(s)
of antibiotics on gastrointestinal tract, 124-125
intraocular pressure, of diluted and new topical corticosteroids, 90-95
of newer drugs, 130-138
side, antibiotic, 140
toxic, specific, drug usage and, 119-126
Eighth nerve damage, 125
Elevation of applanation intraocular pressure
after various dilutions of topical corticosteroids, 92
after various dilutions of topical dexamethasone, 91
Emetine hydrochloride, 150
Endophthalmitis, bacterial, 39
Entamoeba histolytica, 149, 150
Enterobacter, 132
Enzymatic defects in sphingolipidoses, 8
Enzyme activity, excessive, reduction of, in acute intermittent porphyria, 6
Enzymes, 1, 2, 5, 16
Ephedrine, 100, 102
Epidemic keratoconjunctivitis, 78, 83
Epidermophyton floccosum, 145
Epinephrine, 33, 37, 40, 103
and pilocarpine instillation, difference in pressure and outflow facility after, 103
Errors, inborn; *see* Inborn errors
Erythrocin; *see* Erythromycin
Erythromycin, 50, 52, 118, 125, 127, 128, 137, 140, 143
Escherichia coli, 129, 132, 135, 139, 142
Eserine salicylate, 38
Esotropia, 33
Estrogen, 5
Eucatropine, 102
Evaluation, immunologic, of corneal disease, 79
Events, chemical, block of chain of, within cell, 1
Expanders, plasma; *see* Plasma expanders

F

Fabry's disease, 17

Female sex hormones, 5
Fibrinogen, 56
Fibrinolysin, 57, 59-60, 63
Floropryl; *see* Isoflurophate
Food and Drug Administration, 137
Formation and dissolution, thrombus, initiating mechanisms of, 55-56
Formula, structural, of dextran, 57
Fulvicin; *see* Griseofulvin
Fungal disease, agents available for management of, 145-149
Fungi, 81, 82
Fungizone; *see* Amphotericin B
Fusarium, 148

G

Galactose-1-phosphate uridyl transferase, 24, 25, 28
Galactosemia, 24-26
  reduction of substrate or precursors of, 24
  treatment of, 25-26
Gallamine triethiodide, 33
Gamma A antibody, 44
Gamma G antibody, 43
Gamma M antibody, 43
Gangliosides, 10
  Tay-Sachs, 16
Garamycin; *see* Gentamicin
Gastrointestinal disturbance, 124-125
Gastrointestinal tract, effect of antibiotics on, 124-125
Gaucher's disease, 8-13
  biochemical lesion in, 9-10
  diagnosis of, 10-11
  forms of, 9
  genetics of, 9
  treatment of, 11-13
Gene, silent, 97
General pharmacogenetics, 96-97
Gentamycin sulfate, 39, 50, 51, 52, 106, 107, 108, 109, 110, 111, 116, 125, 127, 128, 133, 136-138, 143
Giardia lamblia, 149-150
Glaucoma, 40
Glucocerebrosidase activity, 9-13
Glucocerebroside, 9-10, 12, 27
Glucocorticosteroids, 70, 143
Glucose-6-phosphate dehydrogenase, 97
Glycine, 4
Glycolipid lipidosis, 17
Gonococcus, 79, 80, 84
Griseofulvin, 5, 143, 145

H

Hemoglobin, 4
Hemophilus influenzae, 129
Heparin, 40, 56, 57, 59, 63, 80, 83, 84, 85
Hepatic disease, 4
Hereditary ataxic polyneuritis, 6-7
Herpes infections, prevention of, 43
Herpes keratitis, 43, 44
Herpes simplex, 78, 79, 81, 82, 84, 85, 86, 87
Herpes simplex infections, 43, 44
Herpes zoster, 78, 79, 81, 82
Hexachlorophene, 117
Hexosaminidase-A, 16, 27
High-risk pregnancy, 26
Histamine, 122, 123
Histamine-release testing, 122-123
Histoplasma, 116, 117
Homatropine methylbromide, 40, 102
Homocysteine, 22
Homocystinuria, 22-24
  reduction of substrate or precursors, 24
  therapy for, 23
Hormones, female sex, 5
Hospitals and infection, 113-114
Hydrocortisone, 39, 70, 75, 94
Hydroxyamphetamine, 100
  average increase in pupillary diameter after instillation of, 100
Hydroxypropyl methylcellulose, 39
Hydroxystilbamadine isethionate, 143, 145, 148-149
Hyperemia, conjunctival, 31
Hyperreactivity in Down's syndrome, 33-34
Hypersensitivity, 120, 121
Hypertension, corticosteroid-induced, 90
Hypoglycemic agents, 74
Hypothalamic–pituitary–adrenal gland axis, 73, 74
Hypoxanthine guanine phosphoribosyl transferase, 18
Hypoxantine arabinoside, 47

I

Idoxuridine, 43, 47, 79
IDU; *see* Idoxuridine
Ilotycin; *see* Erythromycin
Immunologic evaluation of corneal disease, 79
Immunosuppressive agents in ophthalmology, 65-67
Imuran; *see* Azathioprine
Inborn errors
  metabolism of, with ocular involvement, management of, 1-28
  of metabolism, categories of, 3-4
  prenatal and neonatal diagnosis of, 2-3
Incidence of intraocular infection, 116-117
Incompatibility, drug, intravenous, 149
Increase

Increase—cont'd
in heart rate after instillation of atropine, 99
in pupillary diameter; *see* Pupillary diameter, increase in
Individual responsiveness to drugs and pharmacogenetics in ophthalmology, 96-103
Infection(s)
agents used to control, 126-129
herpes, prevention of, 43
herpes simplex, 43, 44
hospitals and, 113-114
intraocular
incidence of, 116-117
management of, 138-143
postoperative, 113-117
Infectious corneal disease, corticosteroids in, 77-87; *see also* Corneal disease
Infectious corneal infiltrative diseases, acute, corticosteroid-antimicrobial therapy in, 84-85
Infectious peripheral ischemic syndromes, combined corticosteroid-heparin therapy in, 84
Infiltrative corneal disease, 80-84
Inflammation, recurrent
in corticosteroid-treated cases, 86-87
following combined therapy in infectious central stromal keratitis, 81
following penetrating keratoplasty in infectious central stromal keratitis, 82
and socioeconomic status, correlation between, 82
Influence, racial or pigmentary, on drug responsiveness, 100-103
Influenza vaccination, 44
INH; *see* Isoniazid
Initiating mechanisms of thrombus formation and dissolution, 55-56
Instillation, pilocarpine and epinephrine, difference in pressure and outflow facility after, 103
Instruments, sterilization of, 117
Insulin, 33, 74, 123
Interferon, 44-45, 47
Intraocular infection
incidence of, 116-117
management of, 138-143
Intraocular penetration, 38-40
Intraocular pressure, 37, 98
applanation
elevation of, after various dilutions of topical corticosteroids, 92
of 24 patients after various topical corticosteroids, 92
Intraocular pressure—cont'd
applanation—cont'd
after various dilutions of topical dexamethasone, elevations of, 91
mean applanation, after various corticosteroids, 92, 93
Intraocular pressure effects of diluted and new topical corticosteroids, 90-95
Intraocular pressure responses to topical corticosteroid testing, 97
Intraocular surgery, prophylactic antibiotics for, 138-139
Intravenous drug incompatibility, 149
Involvement, ocular, management of inborn errors of metabolism with, 1-28
Iridocyclitis, 31
Iris cysts, 31
Iritis, 37, 40, 43, 46
Isoflurophate, 30, 31, 32, 33, 34
systemic toxicity of, 32
Isoniazid, 75, 97, 118
Isoprinosine, 46, 47

K

Kanamycin, 39, 111, 118, 125, 127, 128, 136, 140
Kantrex; *see* Kanamycin
Keflex; *see* Cephalexin
Keflin; *see* Cephalothin
Keflordin; *see* Cephaloridine
Keratitis, 40, 43; *see also* Corneal disease
central stromal; *see* Central stromal keratitis
herpes, 43, 44
Keratoconjunctivitis, epidemic, 78, 83
Keratoplasty
combined therapy with, in acute central stromal keratitis, results of, 81
penetrating, 82
in infectious central stromal keratitis, recurrent inflammation following, 82
Klebsiella-aerobacter, 132, 135

L

Lamo; *see* Lanolin, hydrous
Lanolin, hydrous, 121
Lead poisoning, 4
Leishmania donovani, 150
Lens opacities, 31
Lesch-Nyhan syndrome, 18-19
Leuconostoc mesenteroides, 57
Leukocytes, polymorphonuclear, 78, 84
Lidocaine, 50, 51, 79, 80
Lincocin; *see* Lincomycin
Lincomycin, 50, 52, 118, 124, 127, 128, 135-136, 140, 143
Lipid metabolism, 6-18

Lipidoses
  cerebral, 7-8
  glycolipid, 17
Liver disease, 125
Local toxic reactions, 30-31
Long-term patient follow-up of corneal disease, 80
Loridine; *see* Cephaloridine
Lymphocyte transformation test, 123
Lytic agents and plasma expanders in ophthalmology, 55-63

M

Management
  and complications of systemic corticosteroid therapy, 70-76
  of fungal disease, agents available for, 145-149
  of inborn errors of metabolism with ocular involvement, 1-28
  of intraocular infection, 138-143
Matromycin; *see* Oleandomycin
Mean bacterial counts, 109
Measures, therapeutic, for clots, 56-57
Mechanisms
  of action of dextran, 58
  of thrombus formation and dissolution, initiating, 55-56
Medical Letter, 131
Medication, relative cost of, 142-143
Medrysone, 90, 91, 92, 93, 94, 95
  use of, in topical corticosteroid responders, 94
Melarsoprol, 150
Meparacrine hydrochloride, 150
Meperidine, 51
Meprobamate, 5
6-Mercaptopurine, 66, 67, 147
Metabolic defects, heritable, diagnosis of, by amniocentesis, 26-28
Metabolism
  amino acid, 19-24
  categories of inborn errors of, 3-4
  inborn errors of, with ocular involvement, management of, 1-28
  lipid, 6-18
  pigment, 4-6
  sugar, 24-26
Methane sulfonate, 136
Methicillin, 39, 50, 52, 118, 125, 127, 128, 129, 130, 131, 132, 140, 143, 149
Methionine, 22, 23
Methotrexate, 66, 67
Methylprednisolone, 71, 72
Micromonospora purpurea, 111
Microsporum audouini, 145
Microsporum caves, 145
Microsporum gypsum, 145
Microsporum ovale, 145
Miltown; *see* Meprobamate
Mineralocorticoid and antiinflammatory activity of some corticosteroids, comparison of, 71
Miosis, 31
Miotics, strong, toxicity of, in children, 30-34
"Miotic-URI," 34
Mixture, antibiotic-steroid, 54
Modes of therapy for inborn errors, 2
Monilia, 144
Monosialoceramide trihexoside, 16
Moraxella, 78, 81
Movements and preparation of operating team, 117
6-MP; *see* 6-Mercaptopurine
Mucor, 144
Multiplication, bacterial, 105-106
Mycifradin; *see* Neomycin
"Mycobacteria kansasii," 144
Mycobacterium fortuitum, 144, 145
Mycobacterium tuberculosis, 144, 145
Mydriatic administration, topical, average increase in pupillary diameter after, 101
Mydriatics, 36, 40
Myoglobin, 4

N

Nafcillin, 118, 129, 131, 132, 140
Names, trade, and tablet size of some corticosteroids, 71
National Institutes of Health, 66
Naturetics, 72
Neomycin sulfate, 50, 51, 52, 54, 79, 84, 106, 111, 115, 125, 128, 136
Neomycin–polymixin-B–gramicidin ointment, 107, 108, 109, 110
Neonatal and prenatal diagnosis of inborn errors, 2-3
Neosporin; *see* Neomycin
Niemann-Pick disease, 13-15
  biochemical lesion of, 13-14
  diagnosis of, 14-15
  treatment of, 15
  types of, 14
Nocardia asteroides, 144, 146
Nonchromogens, 144
Novobiocin, 118, 125, 127, 128, 137
Nutramigen, 25
Nystatin, 80, 84, 143, 145

O

Observation, daily, 53-54
Occlusion, 55

Occlusion—cont'd
retinal artery, 60-62
Ocular involvement, management of inborn errors of metabolism with, 1-28
Oleandomycin, 125
Opacities, lens, 31
Operating team, preparation and movements of, 117
Ophthalmic solutions, preservatives for, 115
Ophthalmology
immunosuppressive agents in, 65-67
individual responsiveness to drugs and pharmacogenetics in, 96-103
pharmacogenetics in, 97-103
plasma expanders and lytic agents in, 55-63
problems in use of antibiotics in, 113-151
Organ replacement, 13
Osteoporosis, 74-75
Outflow facility and pressure, difference in, after pilocarpine and epinephrine instillation, 103
Oxacillin, 118, 125, 127, 129, 130-131, 132, 140, 143

P

Pannus, 78, 84, 86
Para-aminosalicylic acid, 118
Para-hydroxybenzoates, 115
Paramethasone, 71, 72
Paredrine; *see* Hydroxyamphetamine
Pars planitis, 40
Patients with corneal disease, selection of, 78-79
Patterns of therapy in corneal disease, 79-80
Penbritis; *see* Ampicillin
Penetrating keratoplasty, 82
Penicillin, 50, 51, 114, 118, 120, 121, 123, 126, 128, 129, 130, 131, 132, 133, 134, 135, 138, 140, 143, 146
penicillinase-resistant semisynthetic, choice of, 131-132
repository, 39
water-soluble, 38
Penicillin G, 39, 50, 52, 80, 126, 127, 128, 129, 130, 131, 140, 149
Penicillinase-resistant semisynthetic penicillin, choice of, 131-132
Penicillinic acid, 121
Penicillium, 146
Penicilloyl-polylysine, 122
Penicilloyl-polypeptide compound, 121
Penspek; *see* Phenbenicillin
Pentamidine, 150
Peptic ulcer, 74
Peripheral ischemic or corneal disease, treatment of, 85-86
Pharmacogenetics
and drugs in ophthalmology, individual responsiveness to, 96-103
general, 96-97
in ophthalmology, 97-103
Phenbenicillin, 129
Phenethicillin, 129
Phenyl ethyl alcohol, 115
Phenylalanine, 19-20
Phenylephrine hydrochloride, 31, 40
Phenylketonuria, 19-20
Phenylmercuric nitrate, 115
Photochromagens, 144
Phytanic acid, 6, 7, 27
Pigment metabolism, 4-6
Pigmentary or racial influence on drug responsiveness, 100-103
Pilocarpine, 103
and epinephrine instillation, difference in pressure and outflow facility after, 103
Pimaricin, 85
Plasma, 57
Plasma expanders, 57-59
and lytic agents in ophthalmology, 55-63
Plasma pseudocholinesterase, 32
Plasmin, 59
Plasminogen, 59
Plasmodium, 150
Platelet agglutination, 56
Pneumococci, 135, 139, 142
Pneumococcus, 78, 81
Points in treatment of bacterial corneal ulcers, 48-54
diagnosis of, 49-50
treatment of, 50-54
Poisoning, lead, 4
Polio vaccine, 43
Polymorphonuclear leukocytes, 78, 84
Polymyxin B sulfate, 39, 50, 52, 54, 115, 116, 118, 124, 125, 128, 136, 149
Polyneuritis, hereditary ataxic, 6-7
Porphobilinogen, 4, 5
Porphyria, 4-6
acute intermittent, reduction of excessive enzyme activity in, 6
Porphyria erythropoietica, 4-5
Porphyria hepatica, acute intermittent type, 5-6
Postoperative bacterial counts compared to preoperative counts, 109
Postoperative infection, 113-117
Potassium citrate, 126
Potassium depletion, 75
Potassium iodide, 146
Pralidoxime chloride, 40

Precursors, substrate or, reduction of
in galactosemia, 24
in homocystinuria, 24
in Refsum's disease, 7
Prednisolone, 71, 72, 79
Prednisone, 71, 72, 73, 75, 90
Pregnancy, high-risk, 26
Prenatal and neonatal diagnosis of inborn errors, 2-3
Preparation and movements of operating team, 117
Preservatives, 114-115
for ophthalmic solutions, 115
Pressure and outflow facility, difference in, after pilocarpine and epinephrine instillation, 103
Prevention of herpes infection, 43
Probenecid, 137
Problems in use of antibiotics in ophthalmology, 113-151
Procaine, 37, 121
Programs, screening, 3
Prophylactic antibiotics for intraocular surgery, 138-139
Prophylaxis, antibiotic, 105-111
Propicillin, 129
Propionic acid, 143
Propranolol hydrochloride, 100
Prostaphlin; *see* Oxacillin
Proteus, 34, 114, 124, 129, 132, 136, 139, 142
Proteus mirabilis, 135
Proteus vulgaris, 110
Protopam; *see* Pralidoxime chloride
Pseudocholinesterases, 96
Pseudomonas, 50, 54, 78, 79, 81, 84, 85, 111
Pseudomonas aeruginosa, 114, 117, 124, 129, 132, 136, 137, 139, 142
Pseudomonas pyocyanea, 132, 133
Pupillary block, 31
Pupillary diameter, increase in
after instillation of atropine, 99
after instillation of hydroxyamphetamine, 100
after topical mydriatic administration, 101
Pyopen; *see* Carbenicillin
Pyridoxine, 23
Pyridoxine deficiency, 6
Pyrimethamine, 150

Q

Quaternary ammonium, 116
Quinacrine hydrochloride, 137

R

Racial or pigmentary influence on drug responsiveness, 100-103
Reactions
adverse, 30-33
local toxic, 30-31
Recurrence of acute infectious peripheral corneal disease, 83
Red thrombus, 56, 58
Reduction
of excessive enzyme activity in acute intermittent porphyria, 6
of substrate or precursors
in galactosemia, 24
in homocystinuria, 24
in Refsum's disease, 7
Refsum's disease, 6-7
reduction of substrate or precursors in, 7
Relative cost of medication, 142-143
Renal toxicity, 125-126
Replacement, organ, 13
Repository penicillins, 39
Resistant staphylococci, 140-141
Responses, intraocular pressure, to topical corticosteroid testing, 97
Responsiveness
corticoid, 97-98
drug, racial or pigmentary influence on, 100-103
individual, to drugs and pharmacogenetics in ophthalmology, 96-103
Results of combined therapy
in acute central stromal keratitis, 81
in acute infectious peripheral corneal disease, 83
with keratoplasty in acute central stromal keratitis, 81
Retinal artery occlusion, 60-62
Retinal detachment, 31
Ristocetin, 39
RNA, 2, 12, 45
Route of drug administration, 126

S

Sabin vaccine, 43
Salicylic acid, 143
Saline, 57
Salmonella, 129
Scleritis, 37
Scotochromogens, 144
Screening programs, 3
Selection of patients with corneal disease, 78-79
Selenium sulfide, 145
Serologic testing, 122
Seromycin; *see* Cycloserine
Serum glutamic oxaloacetic transaminase, 130, 131
Serum penicillin, 123
Shelley basophilic degranulation test, 120

Shigella, 129
Side effects, antibiotic, 140
Silent gene, 97
Skin disinfection, 115
Skin testing, 121-122
Smears of corneal ulcers, 49
Socioeconomic status and recurrent inflammation, correlation between, 82
Sodium bicarbonate, 126
Sodium chloride, 80
Sodium desoxycholate, 146
Sodium diphenylhydantoin, 5
Sodium phosphate, 146
Sodium stibogluconate, 150
Sodium sulfacetamide, 138
Solutions
  of antibiotics, concentrated, for topical use, 51-53
  ophthalmic, preservatives for, 115
Sphingolipidoses, 7
  enzymatic defects in, 8
Sphingomyelin, 13, 14, 27
Sphingomyelinase activity, 14-15
Sphingosine, 7
Staphcillin; *see* Methicillin
Staphylococci, 38, 110, 116, 117, 129, 135, 139, 141
  resistant, 140-141
Staphylococcus albus, 114
Staphylococcus aureus, 78, 79, 81, 83, 84, 87, 114, 117, 124, 131, 136, 139, 142
Staphylococcus epidermidis, 78
Status, socioeconomic, and recurrent inflammation, correlation between, 82
Sterilization of instruments, 117
Steroids, 40, 54, 73, 98, 144, 148
  use of, 141-142
Strabismus, 31
Streptococci, 135, 139
Streptococcus, β-hemolytic, 78, 79, 80, 81
Streptokinase, 57, 59, 60, 63
Streptomyces nodosus, 146
Streptomycin, 39, 50, 52, 111, 114, 118, 125, 128, 137, 138, 143
Structural formula of dextran, 57
Study, effectiveness, of antibiotics, 105-111
Subconjunctival antibiotics, 50-51
Subconjunctival repository corticosteroids, 36, 37, 40
Subconjunctival therapy, 36-40
  advantages of, 36
  disadvantages of, 37
  techniques of, 37-38
Substances, chemotherapeutic and antibiotic, toxicity of, 118-119
Substrate or precursors, reduction of; *see* Reduction of substrate or precursors
Succinate, 4
Succinylcholine chloride, 32, 96
Sucrose, 57
Sugar metabolism, 24-26
Sulfacetimide, 107, 108, 109, 110
Sulfadiazine, 127, 146
Sulfanilic acid, 121
Sulfonamides, 118, 120, 121, 123, 126, 137, 146, 150
Suramin sodium, 150
Surgery, intraocular, prophylactic antibiotic for, 138-139
Syndrome
  Down's; *see* Down's syndrome
  infectious peripheral ischemic, combined corticosteroid-heparin therapy in, 84
  Lesch-Nyhan, 18-19
Systemic antifungal agents, 145-149
Systemic corticosteroid therapy, management and complications of, 70-76
Systemic toxicity, 31-32
  of isoflurophate and echothiophate, 32

T

T. microdentium, 137
Tablet size and trade names of some corticosteroids, 71
Tay-Sachs disease, 15-17
  chemistry of, 16
Tay-Sachs ganglioside, 16
Team, operating, preparation and movements of, 117
TegoPen; *see* Cloxacillin
Terramycin; *see* Tetracycline
Test
  lymphocyte transformation, 123
  Shelley basophilic degranulation, 120
Testing
  histamine-release, 122-123
  serologic, 122
  skin, 121-122
  topical corticosteroid, intraocular pressure responses to, 97
Tetracycline, 39, 51, 80, 118, 120, 124, 125, 127, 128, 137, 140, 143, 149
Tetrahydrotriamcinolone, 90
Therapeutic dosage, daily, of corticosteroids, 72
Therapeutic measures for clots, 56-57
Therapy
  combined
    in acute central stromal keratitis, results of, 81
    in acute infectious peripheral corneal disease, results of, 83
    in infectious central stromal keratitis, recurrent inflammation following, 81

Therapy—cont'd
  combined—cont'd
    with keratoplasty in acute central stromal keratitis, results of, 81
  combined corticosteroid-heparin, in infectious peripheral ischemic syndromes, 84
  in corneal disease, patterns of, 79-80
  corticosteroid, systemic, management and complications of, 70-76
  corticosteroid-antimicrobial, in acute infectious corneal infiltrative diseases, 84-85
  modes of, for inborn errors, 2
  subconjunctival, 36-40; *see also* Subconjunctival therapy
  virus, 43-47
Thiazides, 72, 75
Thrombolysin, 59
Thrombophlebitis, 125
Thrombosis, therapies for, 56-57
Thrombus
  red, 56, 58
  white, 56
Thrombus formation and dissolution, initiating mechanisms of, 55-56
Tilorone hydrochloride, 45-46
Tinactin; *see* Tolnaftate
Tolnaftate, 143, 145
Topical anesthetics, 49
Topical use, concentrated solutions of antibiotics for, 51-53
Toxic effects, specific, drug usage and, 119-126
Toxicity
  of antimicrobial agents, 118
  of chemotherapeutic and antibiotic substances, 118-119
  renal, 125-126
  of strong miotics in children, 30-34
  systemic, 31-32
    of isoflurophate and echothiophate, 32
Toxocara canis, 150
Toxoplasma, 150
Trachoma–inclusion conjunctivitis, 78, 79, 80, 83
Trade names and tablet size of some corticosteroids, 71
Treatment
  of bacterial corneal ulcers, points in, 48-54; *see also* Points in treatment of bacterial corneal ulcers
  of peripheral ischemic or corneal disease, 85-86
Triamcinolone, 71, 72, 75
Trichophyton mentagrophytes, 145
Trichophyton rubrum, 145
Trichophyton tonsurans, 145
Trifluorothymidine, 47
Triton X-100, 106
Trypanosoma, 150
d-Tubocurarine, 33
Tyrosine, 20, 21

U

Ulcers
  bacterial corneal, points in treatment of, 48-54; *see also* Points in treatment of bacterial corneal ulcers
  corneal, smears of, 49
  peptic, 74
Undecylenic acid, 143
Unipen; *see* Nafcillin
Uridine diphosphate galactose-4-epimicrase, 25
Urokinase, 57, 59, 60-62, 63
Uroporphyrin, 4, 5
Usage, drug and specific toxic effects, 119-126
Use
  of amphotericin B in chorioretinitis, 147-148
  of medrysone in topical corticosteroid responders, 94
  of steroids, 141-142
  topical, concentrated solutions of antibiotics for, 51-53

V

Vaccination, influenza, 44
Vaccine
  polio, 43
  Sabin, 43
Vancocin; *see* Vancomycin
Vancomycin, 118, 125, 127, 140-141, 149
Vinactane; *see* Viomycin
Viomycin, 118
Virus therapy, 43-47
Visual acuity, 80, 87
Volutella, 148

W

Water-soluble penicillin, 38
White thrombus, 56

X

Xylocaine; *see* Lidocaine

Y

Year Book of Ophthalmology, 138